# Discover & Explore Toronto's Waterfront

A Walker's Jogger's Cyclist's Boater's Guide to
Toronto's Lakeside Sites and History

## Mike Filey

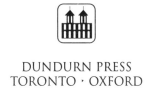

DUNDURN PRESS
TORONTO · OXFORD

Editor: Barry Jowett
Designer: Erich Falkenberg
Printer: Webcom

Canadian Cataloguing in Publication Data

Filey, Mike, 1941-
    Discover & explore Toronto's waterfront: a walker's jogger's cyclist's boater's guide to Toronto's lakeside sites and history

Rev. ed.
Previously published under title: A walker's, jogger's, cyclists's, boater's guide to Toronto's waterfront
ISBN 1-55002-304-7

1. Waterfronts — Ontario — Toronto — Guidebooks.    2. Toronto (Ont.) — Guidebooks.
3. Toronto Islands (Ont.) — Guidebooks.
I. Title.    II. Title: Walker's, jogger's, cyclist's, boater's guide to Toronto's waterfront.

FC3097.18.F54 1998        917.13'541044        C98-931512-6
F1059.5.T683F54 1998

1  2  3  4  5  BJ  02  01  00  99  98

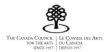

THE CANADA COUNCIL   LE CONSEIL DES ARTS
FOR THE ARTS       DU CANADA
SINCE 1957         DEPUIS 1957

We acknowledge the support of the **Canada Council for the Arts** for our publishing program. We also acknowledge the support of the **Ontario Arts Council** and the **Book Publishing Industry Development Program** of the **Department of Canadian Heritage**.

Care has been taken to trace the ownership of copyright material used in this book. The author and the publisher welcome any information enabling them to rectify any references or credit in subsequent editions.

Printed and bound in Canada.

Printed on recycled paper.

| Dundurn Press | Dundurn Press | Dundurn Press |
| --- | --- | --- |
| 8 Market Street | 73 Lime Walk | 250 Sonwil Drive |
| Suite 200 | Headington, Oxford | Buffalo, NY |
| Toronto, Ontario, Canada | England | U.S.A. 14225 |
| M5E 1M6 | OX3 7AD | |

# Contents

For Holly and her soon-to-be new friend.

Special thanks to Michelle Dale, archivist at the Toronto Harbour Commission, Julie Kirsh and her colleagues at the Toronto Sun News Research Centre, and the people at the Toronto Economic Development Corporation (TEDCO).

All photos are taken from the author's collection.
Maps drawn by Jeff Rickert.

# Preface

I self-published a variation of this guide book a decade ago. Interest in it was considerable and, thankfully, the work was soon out-of-print. With the passage of time, the book has become seriously outdated with many of the buildings no longer there and once-empty spaces now covered with new structures. For those who have the first edition, not to worry; the historical facts remain unchanged.

As far as I was concerned the ever-increasing activity along the water's edge as well as the increased numbers of people visiting the waterfront or, indeed, living there, simply meant that the guide book still had a purpose and, hopefully, sales potential, though this time I would approach a proper publisher. Thus it is that Dundurn Press, which has published all of my recent titles, is on the hook for this one.

In addition to being a guide book of the standard "what's that over there" variety, I have included references to "what *was* that over there" as well as "what *will* be over there." Because of the continuing evolution of Toronto's waterfront that latter question is a particularly difficult one to answer without a crystal ball. Nevertheless, where ideas are firm, or as firm as their spokespersons will admit, I've included them. With Toronto being a living, breathing entity, and thankfully so, there's little doubt that a decade from now this version of the guide will be as dated as my first effort. But for now, have fun, and I hope you learn something about one of the most fascinating places in my city.

\*   \*   \*   \*   \*

NOTE: On June 9, 1998 Royal Assent was given to federal legislation that would create a new Port Authority of Toronto. This new body will replace the Toronto Harbour Commission effective January 1, 1999. The new Authority, similar to sixteen others operating across the country, will have a board consisting of seven members with one member each selected by the federal, provincial, and municipal governments and four by the Toronto business community. This differs from the Toronto Harbour Commission version (established in 1911) that included five commissioners, three of whom were municipal appointments (latterly all elected officials) with the remaining members appointed by the federal government with one of those endorsed by the local board of trade.

# Suggested Reading

While this book is chock full of facts, figures, and, hopefully, fun, I would like to draw attention to a couple of other publications that will further enhance the reader's knowledge and appreciation of Toronto's, and Lake Ontario's, ever-changing waterfront:

*The Waterfront Trail*
(Waterfront Regeneration Trust, 1996)
*More Than an Island* by Sally Gibson
(Irwin Publishing, 1984)
*Trillium and Toronto Island* by Mike Filey
(Peter Martin Associates, 1976)
*I Remember Sunnyside* by Mike Filey
(Dundurn Press, 1996)
*The Great Toronto Bicycling Guide* by Elliot Katz
(Great North Books, 1995)
*The Beach in Pictures 1793–1932* by Mary Campbell and
Barbara Myrvold
(Toronto Public Library, 1988)
*Historical Walking Tour of Kew Beach* by Mary Campbell
and Barbara Myrvold
(Toronto Public Library Board, 1995)

# Introduction

When John Graves Simcoe, the province's first lieutenant-governor and the founder of our city, sailed through the old Western Gap and into the harbour on May 2, 1793, one of the things on his mind was how to keep the pesky Americans he had fought against in the recent war (called either the Revolutionary War or the War of Independence, depending on which team you were cheering for) from overrunning his new province. This concern resulted in the establishment of a naval shipyard at the east end of the harbour. His need to defend the shipyard and the small community of artisans and their families that developed on the nearby shoreline was to result in changes to the waterfront — changes in the form of a pallisaded fort, a pair of unpretentious wooden Parliament Buildings, storehouses, wharves, and some additional buildings in which to house his (and King George III's) loyal subjects who continued to arrive on the now altered shoreline of the new community. Thus, from Toronto's very inception, changes to the waterfront have been part of the city's ongoing development.

In the city's formative years, 1793 to 1850, decisions as to who could do what with lands along the waterfront were left pretty much up to the property owners themselves. It doesn't take a rocket scientist to figure out who those decisions favoured. And while the colonial government did legislate some controls those same officials had many other provincial matters on their collective minds. In addition, what rules they did concoct were usually enforced haphazardly at best and not always with concerns for the city's future in mind. In 1850, it was obvious that a change in the way people thought about the harbour was necessary. Control was placed in the hands of an assortment of officials, some representing the city government, others the newly created harbour commission. Other members looked after the interests of the owners of the newly arrived steam railways (regarded as the "wonder of the age") with a couple of not-totally dispassionate business types thrown in for good measure. The results were both predictable and chaotic. The impact on Toronto's waterfront became apparent as wharves, slips, sewers, industrial sites, train tracks, and rail crossings began to cover virtually every inch of available space from Dufferin Street on the west to Ashbridge's Bay on the east. To say the situation was a mess is an understatement of fearful proportions.

In a bold move to rescue the city's waterfront from total oblivion, in 1911 the federal government created a new harbour commission that submitted to city council the following year an all-encompassing plan that promoted acres and acres of new parkland at the eastern and western extremities of the city (today's Beach and Sunnyside districts, respectively), a magnificent Boulevard Drive (partially realized in Lake Shore Boulevard West), and the creation of industrial and commercial sites along the shoreline of the central and eastern sections of Toronto Harbour. Without question, the parkland at Sunnyside as well as the promised commercial and industrial components were realized. Unfortunately, the 350-acre waterfront park proposed for the stretch of waterfront between the Eastern Channel to well east of Ashbridge's Bay, shall we say, missed the boat. Some damage control was done in later years with the creation of Tommy Thompson Park and public spaces at Ashbridge's Bay Park and Woodbine Beach. In all, the Toronto Harbour Commission, through a series of massive landfilling projects carried out over many years, created new land along the water's edge that would be equivalent to that portion of Toronto bounded by University Avenue, Dundas, Jarvis, and Front streets. Alterations to the waterfront understandably slowed during the war years, but were revived in the 1950s. In the following decade, the vision of high rises all along the central waterfront section began to materialize. Some of the proposed stuctures would go up on a 12-acre (4.8-hectare) parcel of land between Yonge and York streets that years earlier had been proposed as a public park that could have been, as one scribe touted, "a beautiful entrance to the city."

Then came 1972 and the pre-election "gift" of something that would be called Harbourfront (among other things). It was a concept that outgrew its britches.

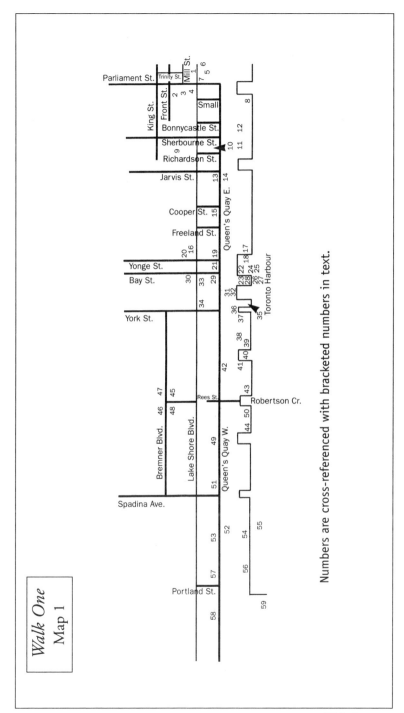

Walk One
Map 1

Parliament St.
Trinity St.
Mill St.
King St.
Front St.
Small
Bonnycastle St.
Sherbourne St.
Richardson St.
Jarvis St.
Cooper St.
Freeland St.
Yonge St.
Bay St.
Queen's Quay E.
Toronto Harbour
York St.
Bremner Blvd.
Lake Shore Blvd.
Rees St.
Robertson Cr.
Queen's Quay W.
Spadina Ave.
Portland St.

Numbers are cross-referenced with bracketed numbers in text.

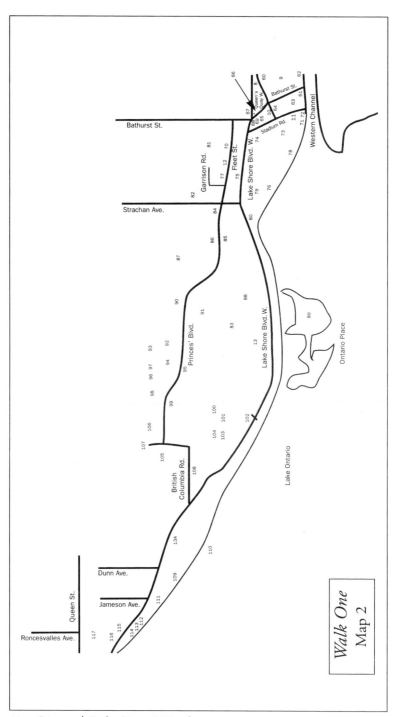

Bathurst St.

Garrison Rd.

Fleet St.

Lake Shore Blvd. W.

Strachan Ave.

Princes' Blvd.

Lake Shore Blvd. W.

British Columbia Rd.

Ontario Place

Lake Ontario

Western Channel

Bathurst St.

Stadium Rd.

Queen's Quay W.

Dunn Ave.

Jameson Ave.

Queen St.

Roncesvalles Ave.

*Walk One*
Map 2

66
67
8
60
9
62
64
65
69
68
10
63
61
11
72
71
73
78
74
81
70
12
77
75
79
76
80
82
84
85
86
87
90
91
88
83
13
89
95
94
92
93
97
96
98
99
101
100
104
103
102
107
106
105
108
13A
110
109
111
117
115
116
114
113
112

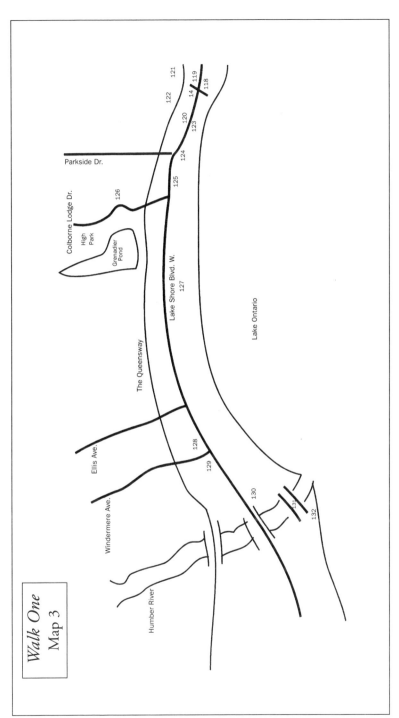

Walk One
Map 3

Parkside Dr.

Colborne Lodge Dr.

High
Park

Grenadier
Pond

The Queensway

Lake Shore Blvd. W.

Lake Ontario

Ellis Ave.

Windermere Ave.

Humber River

121
122
14
119
118
120
123
124
125
126
127
128
129
130
131
132

# Walk One

## Gooderham & Worts to Palace Pier

While we really could start this tour of Toronto's waterfront virtually anywhere along the 12-mile (18-kilometre) stretch between the Humber River to the west and the R.C. Harris Water Treatment plant to the east, I've chosen to begin our tour close to where it all began more than two centuries ago — in fact, at one of the most historic, and least known, intersections in Toronto, the corner of Mill and Trinity streets. In our community's earliest days, this intersection was a mere stone's throw from the water's edge. Over the years numerous landfilling projects have pushed the waters of Toronto Bay further and further south so that today the old corner stands high and dry. Nearby could be found the first Parliament Buildings, the first major industry (see 1) and some of the Town of York's (Toronto's name until city status was achieved in 1834) first residences.

TRINITY STREET: So named for Little Trinity Church at the southwest corner of Trinity and King streets. The church was built in 1843 and today is the oldest church building in the city. One of the benefactors of this historic church was George Gooderham, a co-founder of the Gooderham and Worts distilling company.

MILL STREET: Shortened from the original Windmill Street, so named for its proximity to the original Worts and Gooderham windmill.

\* \* \* \* \*

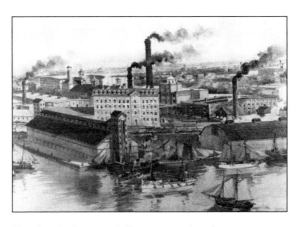

The Gooderham and Worts complex from an 1896 lithograph. The white stone structure still stands.

GOODERHAM AND WORTS LIMITED, 55 Mill Street (1). Until its closing on August 31, 1990, this company was recognized as Toronto's oldest industry in continuous operation. It had been a part of the Toronto scene since 1832. One year earlier, James Worts had arrived in York, as Toronto was then called, looking for a place where he and his brother-in-law, William Gooderham, who had remained in England, could establish for themselves a new business enterprise. Worts decided on a milling operation and soon thereafter, William, accompanied by a contingent of family members, arrived in York to help with the new venture, which was originally known as Worts and Gooderham. By the end of 1832, a large four-vaned Dutch-style windmill, complete with several grinding stones, had been erected on the water's edge so that wheat brought by local farmers could be ground into flour. This windmill was located approximately 250 feet (76.2 metres) south of the main gate, stood over 70 feet (21.3 metres) in height and became a prominent feature of the young city's waterfront. The so-called "Windmill Line," an imaginary line that connected the old windmill with a point of land due south of the old French fort at the foot of today's Dufferin Street in the Exhibition Grounds, was created to define the southerly limit of any and all piers and wharves built out into Toronto Bay. Throughout the 19th century, this Windmill Line was realigned further and further south reflecting the continuous development of the inner harbour. In 1837, following five very successful years in the milling business, Messrs. Worts and Gooderham decided to shift operations slightly and go into the distilling and malting business. Following the tragic suicide death of Worts in 1834, William Gooderham took charge, brought young James

Gooderham Worts into the company, and renamed the enterprise Gooderham and Worts. Within a couple of decades, Gooderham and Worts had become the largest distillery in the world and their products were known and sold far and wide. In 1924 the company was acquired by Hiram Walker Limited of Walkerville, Ontario. In the company's latter years, distilling operations changed from the production of rye whiskey to rum. Molasses, purchased in the West Indies, was transported by tanker at the Port of New York, then barged through the Erie Canal and across Lake Ontario to the Gooderham and Worts dock at the foot of Parliament Street. From here it was pumped to huge storage tanks just west of the distillery building from which it was drawn as needed to manufacture "Maraca" and "Government House" brands of rum. Today, the oldest structures on the site are the two buildings with large green cupolas on their roofs. Both were erected 1858. At the south end of the property stands the white distillery building constructed of Kingston, Ontario, limestone in 1859–60. Following a major fire in October of 1869, the wooden interior of this stone building was destroyed, however the massive outer walls withstood the conflagration. The historic structure was quickly rebuilt and remains an important component of the soon-to-be redeveloped Gooderham and Worts complex. Plans call for a major conversion of the site to mixed uses including housing, retail markets of various types, and museums devoted to children's activities and the history of distilling. The first two residential conversions are presently (July, 1998) under construction on Mill Street east of Trinity and at the Mill and Parliament corner.

## Proceed south on Parliament Street

PARLIAMENT STREET: So named for the first Parliament Buildings in York that were erected on the west side of today's Parliament Street several hundred feet south of Front (see 2) under orders given by the community's founder and the province's first lieutenant-governor, John Graves Simcoe. The upper reaches of this street led to the governor's summer retreat, Castle Frank (named after Simcoe's son Francis) which was located not far from the present subway station of that name. At the lower end of Parliament Street is the Caroline Co-operative housing project. Caroline was the original name given to Sherbourne Street south of Queen Street by the city's founder, Governor John Simcoe, and was meant to honour Caroline, Princess of Wales, later the wife of England's King George IV.

FIRST PARLIAMENT BUILDINGS (site of, 2): West of Parliament Street, just south of the Front Street corner, stood the Parliament Buildings for the Province of Upper Canada. Constructed in 1796 the "complex" consisted of two brick structures, each 40 feet x 25 feet (12 metres x 7.6 metres). The site is now marked by a provincial plaque. The fact that some referred to the unpretentious buildings as the "Palace of Government" resulted in the stretch of Front Street as far west as Jarvis being called Palace Street, a name that obviously didn't stick. The buildings were destroyed by fire during the occupation of York by American forces in April, 1813. Whether the fire was by accident or on purpose was never determined.

FIRST DUEL IN YORK (site of, 3): On January 3, 1800, a duel was enacted by two prominent citizens of York — Clerk of the Executive Council John Small and Attorney General John White — not far from the Parliament Buildings. This action resulted from White's refusal to apologize to Small for disparaging remarks supposedly made by the former's wife about the latter's wife. Very confusing, but what is known is that as a result of the duel, carried out behind the Parliament Buildings of the day, White was mortally wounded by a bullet and died the following day.

PARLIAMENT STREET RAILWAY VIADUCT UNDERPASS (4): One of nine underpasses built as part of the massive $28,476,172 cross-waterfront railway viaduct program built in conjunction with the city's proposed new Union Station on Front Street West. The viaduct construction project was started in 1925 and the section of the viaduct between Church and Cherry streets was constructed on reclaimed land using four million cubic yards of fill dredged from the bottom of the bay. The Parliament Street underpass was opened to vehicular traffic in October of 1927.

GARDINER EXPRESSWAY: So named for the first chairman of Metropolitan Toronto, Frederick G. Gardiner, who served from 1953 to 1961. Construction of the $105-million project, the first urban expressway in Canada, spanned the years 1957–1964.

LAKE SHORE BOULEVARD EAST: Constructed on reclaimed land as part of the Toronto Harbour Commission's huge waterfront redevelopment project undertaken in the 1920s, the section of this thoroughfare from Bathurst to Cherry streets was originally called Fleet Street (after Fleet Street in London, England). The name was officially changed to Lake Shore Boulevard in 1960.

VICTORY SOYA MILLS LIMITED (site of, 5): Massive elevators were built on this site at the southeast corner of Lake Shore Boulevard and Parliament Street in 1943 by industrialist E.P. Taylor in response to the government's request for help in alleviating the shortage of vegetable oils during the Second World War. His company was originally called Sunsoy

Products and it was here that a new type of vegetable oil (new to Canada, at least) known as soya bean oil, was extracted from soya beans, a crop not widely grown in this country. Initial production volumes were small. Anticipating victories over Germany and Japan, a patriotic Taylor changed the name of the company to Victory Mills with the first delivery of soya beans, 110,000 bushels of them, arriving on board the S.S. *Cheyenne* on July 3, 1945. Over the ensuing years the plant was expanded several times to keep up with the ever-increasing demands. In its heyday Victory Soya Mills, which had become the largest plant of its kind in Canada, processed more than 1,800 tonnes of soya beans a day that had been trucked to the plant from farms in southwestern Ontario or shipped to the site by freighter from Great Lakes ports like Chicago, Illinois and Toledo, Ohio. The processed soya bean meal, oil, and flour, as well as lecithin, a product used in candies, cosmetics, paints, and inks, were shipped to markets all over the world. For a variety of financial reasons, it was decided to close this once very busy plant in 1991. The elevator was demolished several years later.

CANADA MALTING (site of, 6): The elevators that are still seen were erected in 1947–48 by a sister company of Victory, Canada Malting. Their future is very uncertain. Uncertain too is the re-use of this prime piece of property now controlled by the Toronto Economic Development Corporation (TEDCO), and while various ideas have been brought forward (housing or large retail stores to mention just two), ongoing litigation will continue to be a major stumbling block to any redevelopment proposal.

REPLICA OF THE GOODERHAM AND WORTS WINDMILL (site of, 7): In 1954, as a civic gesture, the Gooderham and Worts company built a scaled-down version of their historic and long-since-demolished windmill (see 1) at the southeast corner of Fleet (now Lake Shore Boulevard) and Parliament streets, a location almost 1,200 feet (366 metres) southwest of the structure's original location on the distillery property. Construction of the Gardiner Expressway in the late 1950s meant that even the replica had to be demolished.

## Proceed south and west on Queen's Quay

QUEEN'S QUAY EAST: As part of the Toronto Harbour Commission's redevelopment of the Central Harbour Terminal area, a new street called Queen's Quay (pronounced Queen's "key") was opened along the water's edge on land reclaimed from Toronto Bay. The new thoroughfare was built in sections as waterlots were filled in. Queen's Quay now stretches from Parliament Street westerly to Stadium Road. Seen along the street are

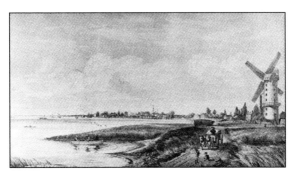

The Gooderham and Worts windmill overlooking Toronto Bay, 1834.

signs indicating the route of the Martin Goodman Trail. This 12-mile (19.5-kilometre) pathway for walkers, joggers, and cyclists is named in honour of a distinguished journalist and former president of the *Toronto Star* newspaper (see 19), and was presented to Toronto on the occasion of the city's 150th birthday in 1984.

ROYAL CANADIAN YACHT CLUB MAINLAND DOCK (8): It is from here that the historic passenger ferries *Hiawatha* and *Kwasind* depart for the RCYC's Island clubhouse (see 176).

SMALL STREET: Though it is now just a small street, this thoroughfare was originally the southernmost part of Berkeley Street to the north. The construction of Lake Shore Boulevard and the railway viaduct in the 1920s resulted in the street being "orphaned." To avoid subsequent confusion the now-isolated street was given a new name. Small honours Major John Small, the first clerk of the new province's executive council and a prominent citizen in York (Toronto's name prior to incorporation as a city on March 6, 1834). On January 3, 1800, John Small shot and killed John White in York's first duel (see 3). Incidently, Berkeley Street, from which Small Street was carved, was named for Berkeley House, which once stood at the southwest corner of today's King and Berkeley streets. Berkeley House, in turn, was named for the birthplace in Gloucestershire, England, of Major Small. So while the streets aren't connected physically, they are historically.

BONNYCASTLE STREET: Another "orphaned" thoroughfare (it was part of Princess Street before the construction mentioned above), Bonnycastle was named in honour of Sir Richard Bonnycastle, who served in Canada with the British forces during the War of 1812. In 1835, as a captain in the Royal Engineers, he wrote a report on the deplorable condition of both Toronto Bay and the marshes in Ashbridge's Bay. In his report he advocated the construction of a canal through the narrows on the Peninsula (now Toronto Island) to permit an increased flow of water in and out of the bay as well as allowing a new passageway for sailing vessels. Little was done to implement Bonnycastle's recommendations, however a violent storm in 1858 caused a permanent breach at the narrows which has since been developed into the East Gap. Bonnycastle's Royal Engineers were also responsible for the construction of the first permanent bridges over the mouths of the Don River in 1835 for which the citizens were extremely grateful, several of them having drowned attempting to cross the waterway in the past. Bonnycastle was appointed as commanding officer of the Royal Engineers in Canada West (Ontario) in 1837 and was subsequently knighted for his services in the defence of Kingston. In 1842, he authored *The Canadas in 1841*, a book in which he described a return visit to Toronto. He commented that while disembarking from his vessel moored at Maitland's Wharf (foot of Church Street) he was "almost jostled into the water by rude carters plying for hire on its narrow bounds while being pestered by crowds of equally rude pliers for hotel preferences."

LOWER SHERBOURNE STREET: Samuel Ridout, whose family was from Sherbourne, Dorsetshire, England, was born in Virginia in 1778 and at the age of 19 emigrated to Canada with his family. He eventually obtained a position in the office of the surveyor-general of Upper Canada in York (now Toronto) and, in 1818, purchased Park Lot 4 for $2,400 from the estate of the late John White, who had been killed in the community's first duel (see 3). This was one of the large one-hundred-acre plots of land laid out by Governor Simcoe, the promise of which the governor used to entice the well-to-do to settle in his new capital in the wilderness. These lots fronted on a pathway blazed through the forest that was simply named Lot Street. We recognize that thoroughfare today as Queen Street. The boundaries of Samuel Ridout's property were the present-day thoroughfares Queen, Seaton, Bloor, and Sherbourne. A few years later, Samuel sold the west half of his property to his half-brother, Thomas Gibbs Ridout, cashier (or general manager) of the prosperous Bank of Upper Canada. In 1857, Thomas started to build a new mansion for himself, a residence he named Sherborne House after the Ridout family home in Sherborne, Dorsetshire, England. Soon, the road leading to Ridout's new residence became known as Sherbourne Street. Today's spelling features an extra letter, "u". Why? No one knows.

To continue the Ridout story, the Bank of Upper Canada folded before he could move into his new residence and Sherborne House had to be sold. After a succession of owners, including H.H. Fudger, president of the

Robert Simpson Company, who converted the house into a residence called Fudger House for some of Simpson's female employees, the stately old building was demolished in 1964. Originally, the stretch of Sherbourne Street south of Queen was given the name Caroline by the city's founder, John Graves Simcoe, to honour Princess Caroline, the wife of England's King George IV.

KNAPP'S ROLLER BOAT (site of, 9). In 1897, Prescott, Ontario lawyer/inventor Frederick Knapp commissioned the Polson Iron Works Company to build a prototype of his creation, a boat that would roll over the top of the water thereby preventing passengers from experiencing seasickness, or so he predicted. The Polson ship yard was located on the water's edge at the foot of Sherbourne Street, a location that today would be many hundreds of feet to the north. As it turned out, the Roller Boat was unsuccessful in its mission and Knapp eventually abandoned his dream and returned to Prescott, leaving the craft moored in Polson's ship yard. Using the rusting shell as landfill, the craft was eventually buried somewhere in the vicinity of today's Lake Shore Boulevard–Sherbourne Street intersection. It's reported that the presence of the buried hulk resulted in a re-alignment of the Gardiner Expressway, since the supports for the overhead highway could not be sunk where originally planned. True? Who knows. But it's a great story.

\* \* \* \* \*

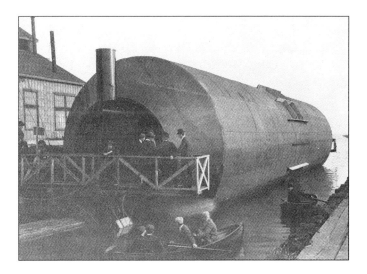

Mr. Knapp's revolutionary (and less-than-successful) Roller Boat, 1897.

FEDERAL EXPRESS WATERFRONT TERMINAL (10). Federal Express Canada Ltd. began work on this 61,500-square-foot state-of-the-art facility to serve the company's downtown customers in 1996. More than 150 employees moved into the building the following year. Federal Express, now the world's largest express transportation company, first went into business south of the border in 1973, moving into Canada in 1987. The company serves 212 countries, moves an average of 2.9 million packages daily worldwide, and has a fleet of 596 planes making FedEx the 9th largest airline in the world.

CINESPACE (11): This mammoth structure was originally built by the Toronto Harbour Commission in anticipation of increased shipping traffic to the Port of Toronto as a result of the recently constructed St. Lawrence Seaway. The first warehouse built to take advantage of the Seaway was Marine Terminal 11, some 100,000 square feet (9,290 square metres) in size. It was erected at the foot of Yonge Street in 1954 and subsequently renamed MT 27. This warehouse was demolished in the 1980s. Two years after Marine Terminal 11 opened construction began on a second facility of similar size at the foot of Jarvis Street followed soon thereafter by a third 100,000-square-foot warehouse just to the east. Together, these new facilities provided a total of 200,000 square feet of storage space under cover with an additional twenty-two acres of outside space. They opened in 1959, the same year that the new Seaway was ready for traffic. It was during the visit of Queen Elizabeth II to Toronto in June, 1959, shortly after she and American president Dwight Eisenhower had jointly opened the Seaway, that what at first had been identified as Marine Terminals 15 and 17 were renamed MT 28 and MT 29, the "Queen Elizabeth Docks." In 1995 the huge building took on a new role, this time as the home of four huge motion picture sound stages ranging in size from 10,000 square feet to 45,000 square feet, the latter being one of the largest on the continent. In addition to the sound stages, the building contains makeup, wardrobe, and dressing rooms, production offices, and catering facilities. Some of the movies produced here include *The Santa Clause*, *Good Will Hunting*, *The Corrupters*, and *The Storm of the Century*. In the latter production a large portion of the interior of this building was converted into a small town in Maine that was caught in the grips of the ice storm that paralyzed parts of eastern Canada and the United States in early 1998.

Returning to the Seaway story for a moment, the original concept of a shipping corridor made up of canals connecting the Great Lakes with the Atlantic Ocean some 2,300 miles (3,700 kilometres) to the east actually goes back as far as 1895 when the American and Canadian governments set up a Deep Waterway Commission. Over the following five decades there was a lot of talking, but nothing really happened until 1951 when the Canadian government established the St. Lawrence Seaway Commission with a mandate to build, operate, and maintain a seaway with, or without, the co-operation of the United States. And, if necessary, that project would be entirely within Canada. At virtually the last moment, the American government decided to join with Canada in the construction of 191 miles (307 kilometres) of canals. Work on the vast project started simultaneously on both sides of the border on August 10, 1954. The St. Lawrence Seaway opened on June 26, 1959.

WATERFRONT TENNIS CLUB (12): In the summer of 1985, two huge air-supported structures situated between MT 28 and MT 29 were inflated and what was originally called the Queen's Quay Racquet Club was in business. Today, there are seven tennis courts as well as two squash courts inside the two "bubbles." The club also features fitness facilities and a public restaurant.

RICHARDSON STREET: This street was named in honour of Captain Hugh Richardson who was born in London, England, in 1789. At the age of nine, Richardson left school and went to sea. While navigating through the English Channel in the seventeenth year of the seemingly endless war between Britain and France, he was captured by a French privateer and imprisoned for eight years. In 1821, Richardson made his way to Canada and two years later joined the Second Militia Regiment, East York, as a captain. Utilizing his knowledge of sailing vessels, he built the steamers *Canada* and *Chief Justice Robinson* of 250 and 400 tons respectively. He also developed an intense interest in the commercial development of Toronto Harbour and in 1837 was appointed one of three Harbour Commissioners along with Major Bonnycastle (see Bonnycastle Street) and Chief Justice Draper. In 1852, Richardson was appointed Harbour Master, a position he held until his death in 1870.

LOWER JARVIS STREET: When Governor Simcoe convened the first meeting of the executive council of his new Province of Upper Canada in the provisional capital of York on September 2, 1793, one of the members, William Jarvis, was still across the lake at the old capital of Newark (now Niagara-on-the-Lake) tidying up his affairs. Jarvis was born in Stamford, Connecticut, in 1756. With hostilities between the States and Great Britain on the horizon, Jarvis, who wanted to remain loyal to his monarch, King George III, joined John Simcoe's Queen's Rangers, a British militia unit. Following hostilities, Jarvis returned to England. Soon his former commanding officer offered him the position of provincial secretary in Simcoe's new area of responsibility, the recently established Province of

Upper Canada. Even though Jarvis wasn't present at Simcoe's inaugural council meeting, the Governor granted him one hundred acres of land on the west of the Don River and fronting on Lot Street (now Queen Street). It was a reward for remaining loyal to the Crown, and to Simcoe. Soon after receiving the grant Jarvis traded his property for one a little further to the west which had originally been given to David Smith, the acting surveyor-general. In 1817, just days before his death, William Jarvis transferred his newly acquired parcel of land to his son Samuel Peters Jarvis. Young Sam had been a combatant in York's second, and last, duel, which took place near the present Bay and College Street intersection on Saturday, July 12, 1817. In fact, he was still in jail on a charge of murder that followed the duel when the news arrived that his father had died. Sam was acquitted of the murder charge (duels, provided they were carried out properly, were still legal in 1817) and twenty years later was appointed to the position of Chief Superintendent of Indian Affairs. After just eight years at this post, he was found guilty of manipulating the department's accounts. It was estimated that Jarvis owed the government more than $20,000, and as a result was dismissed from his post. In an effort to pay some of his debts, Jarvis decided to subdivide and sell off the one-hundred-acre lot his father had given to him. John George Howard, architect, surveyor, and, much later, benefactor of the city's beautiful High Park, was hired and drew up plans for subdividing the property. For easier access to the subdivided lots a thoroughfare was carved northward through the middle of the property. It connected Queen Street with the Concession Road (now Bloor Street) and was named Jarvis Street in tribute to this pioneering Toronto family.

LOBLAWS SUPERMARKET (13): Built on the site of an Ontario Provincial Police garage and Orange Crush bottling plant, this new 78,000-square-foot, three-storey Loblaws supermarket opened in the spring of 1997. Loblaws has an interesting history with Toronto's waterfront, having built a mammoth warehouse facility at the corner of Front and Bathurst streets back in 1927 (see 67). More than just your average supermarket, this complex features:
- a Loblaws grocery store and pharmacy
- an LCBO store
- a Mövenpick Marché restaurant, seating seventy people
- a Club Monaco Everyday store, selling clothing as well as kitchen and bathroom accessories and other products for the home
- a cigar store
- a Moving Store kiosk
- an organic foods store
- a community meeting place

REDPATH SUGARS LIMITED: 95 Queen's Quay East (14): When the St. Lawrence Seaway opened in June of 1959, the first industry in the province to commence operations as a direct result of this new 191-mile (307-kilometre) "canal" was the Redpath Sugar refinery on the Toronto waterfront. (By the way, the name Redpath honours John Redpath, who established Canada's first successful sugar refinery on the Lachine Canal in Montreal in 1854.)

Back to Toronto. Raw sugar, a brown, sticky substance that's shipped to Toronto from sugar plantations around the world, is unloaded at the Redpath dock from large ocean-going ships (the average load is about ten thousand tonnes) using a huge scoop which dumps the sugar mixture onto a conveyor belt which, in turn, directs the raw sugar into the adjacent large A-frame storage building. The processing starts with the raw sugar being directed via trap doors and more conveyor belts to the main processing plant where it is subjected to extensive purification, granulation, and refining operations. The refined sugar is then graded, packaged, and stored prior to shipment by truck and railway car to consumers across the country. Redpath Sugars has a fascinating museum on-site which is well worth a visit. A recent addition to the Queen's Quay facade of the storage building is a huge mural, 97 feet (31.5 metres) high and 146 feet (47.5 metres) wide, created by American artist Wyland. Titled "Whaling Wall" it was number seventy in a series of similar murals across North America that emphasize the importance of preserving ocean environments. The work was created in the fall of 1997.

COOPER STREET: William Cooper settled in York about 1795 and thirteen years later built the town's first substantial wharf at the foot of Church Street. It was at Cooper's Wharf that the first of the large schooners and the first steamers to visit York moored to load or unload passengers and freight. With the landfilling that has taken place over the years, this historic wharf has long since disappeared under the railway tracks to the north of this intersection. Fortunately, Cooper, a man who was important to the early development of Toronto's harbour, has at least been immortalized in the name of this small street.

LIQUOR CONTROL BOARD OF ONTARIO (LCBO) RETAIL STORE, (15): Prohibition came to Ontario in 1916 and for the next eleven years the province was "dry." In 1927, the Ontario Temperance Act was repealed by the Liquor Control Act, and the Liquor Control Board of Ontario (LCBO) was established to regulate the distribution and sale of liquor throughout the province. On June 1 of that year the first sixteen liquor stores opened with six of them here in Toronto. Store No. 1 was at the northeast corner of Church and Lombard streets in a building that still stands. In 1947, the Liquor Licence Board of Ontario was established to grant licences and inspect licenced premises. In September, 1954, both the LCBO and LLBO moved into the building at the north end of this block where today their respective administration facilities are located. In addition, there is a liquor warehouse, a delivery depot, and several bottling lines for the various LCBO brands of liquor in the 55 Lake Shore Boulevard East building. The LCBO liquor store at the corner of Queen's Quay and Cooper Street opened in June of 1952. It has since become the largest liquor store in the country and one of the largest on the continent, offering more than four thousand varieties of liquors and spirits from around the world for sale. In October of 1990, Vintages — the fine wine, spirits, and specialty beer division of the LCBO — opened an outlet in the store. Vintages now offers more than two thousand different wines and liquors. In its selection is Chateau La Fleur, a French bordeaux wine bottled in 1947. At $5,495 (plus tax) it's the most expensive in the store. We've come a long way from the days when customers filled out a slip then waited while a member of the staff retrieved the order from a dark back room. In fact, this liquor store even offers a wine appreciation series (sampling included) and "Tutored Tastings," an opportunity to learn more about the various products and services offered by the LCBO.

FREELAND STREET: Peter Freeland was born in Scotland and emigrated to the States in 1819, moving to Montreal soon thereafter where he established a soap and candle-making factory. About 1832, while Toronto was still the Town of York, he moved here and built a large three-storey factory on the east side of an old wharf located at the foot of Yonge Street. A portion of the factory was built over the water lot that extended east to the foot of Scott Street and south to the Windmill Line (see 1). Here Freeland mixed grease, tallow, and rosin collected from various sources around town in huge kettles with wood ashes and lime. (Occasionally, to keep up with demand, he would have to import tallow from Rochester across the lake.) The reaction produced soap which was then cut into bars and sold. Candles were made in a similar fashion using specially designed candle molds. Peter Freeland died in 1861 and soon, like his soap, the company dissolved. Landfilling operations in the latter half of the last century and the subsequent building of the railway viaduct buried any trace of this early Toronto industry, but its entrepreneurial owner is still remembered in this street name.

\* \* \* \* \*

TORONTO AIR HARBOUR (site of, 16): Long before anyone had thought of a site on the Island or out at Malton as a place to build an airport, the Toronto Harbour Commission developed a small air base at the foot of Scott Street (subsequently renamed Freeland Street) on Toronto's fast changing waterfront. On July 15, 1929, this "temporary" facility was officially opened with a boisterous send-off for a Colonial Airways Sikorsky amphibian aircraft christened *Neekah* (an Amerindian word for goose), which was carrying mail bound for Buffalo, New York. The forty-five-minute flight was timed to connect with the westbound transcontinental night air mail service from that city. This pioneer marine airport went out of business several years later and all traces were buried under the fill used to create new land to the east of the Yonge Street slip.

MARINE TERMINAL 27 (site of, 17): Constructed by the Toronto Harbour Commission in 1954 and originally called Marine Terminal 11, this 100,000-square-foot (9,290-square-metre) facility was the first structure to be built in anticipation of the increased traffic expected in the Port of Toronto following the opening of the proposed St. Lawrence Seaway later in the decade. It was demolished in 1988 and the site awaits redevelopment.

\* \* \* \* \*

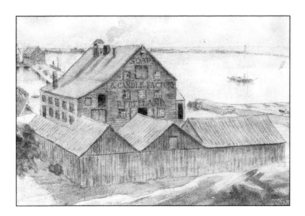

Peter Freeland's soap and candle factory. See Freeland Street.

YONGE STREET: One of the first letters written by John Graves Simcoe, the new lieutenant governor of the Province of Upper Canada, was a short note to his friend and secretary of war in the cabinet of King George III, Sir George Yonge (1732–1812), in which Simcoe stated that "the military roads and communication [in the new province] will require some investigation." The second of these military roads (Dundas Street was first) was completed in 1796 and connected the provisional capital of York with Lake Huron to the north (via the Holland River, Lake Simcoe, etc.) so that in the event of trouble with the Americans (Simcoe hated the Americans and anticipated an invasion of the capital which, in fact, did occur in 1813), troops and stores could be swiftly brought to help defend the provincial capital at York. At first, this military road, which Simcoe named after his friend Yonge, ended abruptly at today's Bloor Street with all traffic entering or leaving York via Yonge having to detour along Bloor to enter or leave the town by way of Parliament Street to the east. In actual fact, a narrow, virtually impassable road did descend south from Yonge as far as today's Queen Street, but because the land south of Queen was swampy and impassable it was little used. In 1802, the section of Yonge between Queen and Bloor Streets had been improved and traffic could now travel, with much difficulty, from the corner of today's Queen and Yonge streets north to Holland Landing. The section of Yonge south of Queen down to the old shoreline wasn't opened for another dozen or so years. Eventually, over many decades, Yonge Street was extended further and further north so that today the street, at 1,178.3 miles (1,896.3 kilometres) is listed in the Guiness Book of World Records as the "longest street in the world." Yonge Street stretches from its intersection with Lake Shore Boulevard a block north of Toronto Bay to its termination at the bridge leading into the State of Minnesota at the western limits of the Northwestern Ontario community of Rainy River. In the pavement on the south side of Queen's Quay is a "mileage chart" of distances to various points along the length of Yonge Street.

CAPTAIN JOHN'S HARBOUR BOAT RESTAURANT, 1 Queen's Quay West (18): "Captain" John Letnik arrived in Toronto from his native Yugoslavia in 1957. Unable to speak a word of English, John had a tough time at first, but eventually obtained work washing dishes in the kitchen at the St. George's Golf and Country Club in Etobicoke. Over the next five years, John saved as much money as possible and soon opened his own thirty-seat restaurant in downtown Toronto. So successful was this venture that he was finally able to take his first real holiday. It was while crossing the Atlantic on the S.S. *France* and enjoying the superb service and delicious meals on board ship that John made the decision to open a floating restaurant somewhere on Toronto's waterfront. John's first harbourfront restaurant was a converted ex-Detroit boat/ex-Georgian Bay ferry that was

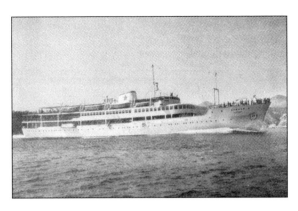

M.S. *Jadran* is now a floating restaurant at the foot of Yonge Street.

introduced to the public at its new Yonge Street berth in 1972. Three years later, John introduced another vessel to Torontonians, the 297-foot (90.5-metre) Mediterranean cruise ship M.S. *Jadran* ("Jadran" is the Yugoslavian word for "Adriatic," the sea between Yugoslavia and Italy). *Jadran* was built in Split, Yugoslavia, in 1957 and operated on the Rijeka-Dubrovnic-Venice route until acquired by Captain John in 1975. Major renovations have converted the ship into a unique one-thousand-seat waterfront restaurant and banquet facility.

TORONTO STAR, 1 Yonge Street (19): Now the most widely read newspaper in Canada, *The Toronto Star* was first published in 1892 as the *Toronto Evening Star* by twenty-one printers and four apprentices who had gone out on strike against the owners of another city newspaper, the *Toronto News*. The *Star's* first edition of eight thousand copies, supplemented by a second edition of two thousand copies, hit the city streets on Thursday, November 3 of that year. Selling for one cent, the *Evening Star* joined the other seven daily newspapers — *Empire, Telegram, World, Mail, Globe*, and the new paper's nemesis, the *News* — that were available to the 150,000 citizens of a city not yet sixty years old. For the first few years the *Star* was assembled in a couple of rooms at 114 Yonge Street and printed on the press of a rival paper. A few years later the paper was put together and printed in the Saturday Night Building at 26–28 Adelaide Street West. Then, under Joseph Atkinson, one of the most influential newspaper people of his day, *The Toronto Star*, as it was now called, moved into its very own building at 18–20 King Street West where it was published for the next twenty-five years. (An interesting sidelight about this latter building is that Canada's first regular daily radio broadcast over the *Star*'s own station, CFCA, emanated from 18–20 King Street West from 1922 until the station moved to a building at the southwest corner of Yonge Street and St. Clair Avenue in 1924, where it continued to broadcast until 1933.) By the mid-twenties, the *Star* had again outgrown its surroundings and a new location was sought. In late 1927, work began on a twenty-three-storey skyscraper further west along King Street into which the paper moved over the February 2–3, 1929, weekend. The new building at 80 King Street West served well until the *Star*, again needing more space, moved to the foot of Yonge Street in 1972. the actual printing of the paper is now done on presses in the Town of Vaughan, north of the city.

YONGE STREET RAILWAY VIADUCT UNDERPASS (20): Looking north up Yonge Street we can see the long underpass that permits both vehicle and pedestrian traffic a safe and quick way of avoiding the multitude of railway tracks that traverse the city's waterfront. But it wasn't always as easy as it is today. In fact, until work was completed on the long-awaited cross-waterfront railway viaduct in the mid-1920s (see 4), pedestrians, horse-drawn wagons, and, eventually, automobile and truck traffic had to cross numerous sets of tracks at grade. Accidents and delays were a regular occurrence. Then, because of the confusion surrounding the final location of tracks into and out of the new Union Station, the completion of the underpasses at Yonge, Bay, and York streets was delayed for years. It wasn't until August 20, 1930, that the Yonge Street underpass we use today finally opened to traffic.

"BETWEEN THE EYES" (21): Located on the northwest corner of Yonge Street and Queen's Quay is this unusual steel and polished steel sculpture by Richard Deacon. Commissioned by Camrost Development Corporation, it was unveiled in 1990.

*LAKE RUNNER* (22): Operated by Shaker Cruise Lines, this 275-passenger vessel runs a frequent eighty-five- to ninety-minute service between its dock here at the foot of Yonge Street and ports on the Niagara peninsula. Constructed in 1984–85 in Georgetown, Prince Edward Island, and launched as *Marine Courier*, the craft originally served various ports along the coast of Newfoundland before being relocated to Toronto and renamed.

WESTIN HARBOUR CASTLE HOTEL, 1 Harbour Square (23): This hotel and the nearby condominium complex to the west are all that remain of an extremely ambitious $100-million redevelopment project first proposed by Leslie Marlowe in the 1962. He envisioned 2,300 apartment units in a series of high-rise towers, a thirty-six-storey office tower, a motor hotel, mercantile centre, ferry docks, and marine terminal. The so-called Marvo project ran out of steam and in 1972 the land was purchased by Ottawa developer/builder Robert Campeau. Soon thereafter work on what was to open as the Toronto Hilton Harbour Castle Hotel began on land reclaimed from Toronto Bay. The hotel eventually came under new ownership and it is now the Westin Harbour Castle Hotel with a total of 974 rooms in two towers of thirty-five floors each. On top of the South Tower is the two-storey Lighthouse revolving restaurant. The first guests in the new luxury hotel arrived in the spring of 1975. Before long, the hotel's Conference Centre on the north side of Queen's Quay (which is connected to the hotel by a glass-encased pedestrian bridge) opened. The centre's largest facility, the Metropolitan Room, can seat up to 2,500.

LAKE STEAMER DOCKS (site of, 24): During the latter part of the nineteenth century and well into the twentieth, the number of passenger steamers operating out of the Port of Toronto was quite staggering. There were daily cruises spring, summer, and fall from Toronto to Niagara-on-the-Lake, Queenston, Lakeside Park (now part of St. Catharines), Hamilton, Oakville, Long Branch, Rochester, the 1000 Islands, and even Montreal. For years, every day during the sailing season Toronto Harbour would be packed with lake steamers with impressive and mysterious names like *Empress of India, Persia, Corsican, Lakeside, Garden City, Toronto, Kingston, Turbinia, Dalhousie City, Northumberland, Modjeska, Macassa, Chippewa, Tionesta, Corona, Chicora, Cayuga,* and the ill-starred *Noronic* (see 25). One of the busiest docks was that of Canada Steamship Lines (CSL). It was located on the south side of Queen's Quay just east of the foot of Bay Street, right where the Westin Harbour Castle Hotel stands today. The $2-million CSL facility was opened in July of 1927 and served hundreds of thousands of excited fun-seekers until economics, and the family automobile, signalled the end of our "love boats." The CSL docks were demolished in 1964 and the slip filled in. A decade later work began on the new Harbour Castle Hotel.

S.S. *NORONIC* DISASTER (site of, 25): Usually found cruising the upper Great Lakes, the magnificent Canada Steamship Lines passenger ship S.S. *Noronic* arrived in Toronto Harbour on the afternoon of Friday, September 16, 1949, for an overnight stay prior to continuing her special early autumn cruise from Detroit and Cleveland to the 1000 Islands. At 2:38 AM Saturday morning, an alarm was received at the Toronto Fire Department's Adelaide Street Station. "Fire at Pier 9!" screamed the message. The trucks rolled, but even as the men arrived just minutes later it was obvious that the huge cruise ship was doomed. There was nothing else to do but play hoses on the inferno and try and get as many people off the blazing ship as possible. The flames were so intense that nearby vessels were smoldering. As the sky lit up and screams pierced the cool evening air, crews rushed to back *Cayuga* and *Kingston* away from their nearby wharves. For hours, men fought the flames while police and other volunteers plucked passengers from the flaming decks of the stricken *Noronic* and from the sizzling water in the slip. The next morning crowds streamed to the waterfront where they saw the once majestic ship lying on her side, capsized by the tons of water poured aboard her to douse the flames that had raced through the paint-encrusted wooden corridors of the once-proud thirty-six-year-old pride of the CSL fleet. The death toll was horrific and continued to grow throughout the days that followed. Charred remains were taken to the Horticultural Building on the Exhibition Grounds for identification. The final count revealed 119 had perished. Many of the unidentified victims were subsequently buried in a mass grave in Toronto's Mt. Pleasant Cemetery. There, a sombre memorial stands as a reminder of what was, and hopefully will always be, our city's worst disaster.

ISLAND FERRY DOCKS (26): For more than a century-and-a-half, Torontonians have travelled to their beloved Island on ferry boats of various shapes and sizes. And during that time numerous schemes that would do away with the so-called "old-fashioned" Island ferries have been brought forward. Bridges for pedestrians and electric streetcars, underwater tunnels, and even aerial tramcars have been suggested. At one point, futuristic magnetic levitation vehicles with linear induction motors operating on "skyways in the air" were seen as the perfect replacement for the ferry boats. While clever ideas such as these come and go, the Island ferries seem to be here forever, much to the delight of Torontonians and visitors alike.

The city's very first ferry boat, introduced in 1833, was a scow-like craft named *Sir John of the Peninsula* (the term "Peninsula" was used since at that time Toronto Island was still connected to the mainland at the east end). The *Sir John* was powered by two horses walking a circular treadmill that was connected to a pair of side-paddles. Soon large numbers of other craft arrived on the bay and before long a ferry boat service was being provided from wharves scattered all along the waterfront in a less-than-satisfactory manner by a multitude of private operators. Then, in 1890, the Toronto Ferry Company (TFC) was created and absorbed these smaller companies. The company provided service to Ward's Island, Island Park, and Hanlan's Point from its dock at the foot of Bay Street until ferry service became publicly owned in 1927. In that year, the Toronto Transportation Commission (TTC), which had been busily operating streetcars and buses on the city streets since 1921, added ferry boats to their fleet. The TTC immediately consolidated ferry boat operations in a new mainland terminal building on the south side of Queen's Quay just west of the foot of Bay

Street. Here the big red cars of the TTC would drop off thousands of eager and happy Island visitors every spring, summer, and fall. In 1972, as part of the redevelopment of the waterfront at the foot of Yonge Street, a new ferry terminal was incorporated into the new hotel project. The entrance to the terminal is on the west side of the hotel where the double-end diesel-powered ferries *William Inglis, Thomas Rennie, Sam McBride*, the smaller *Ongiara*, and the steam-powered *Trillium*, are berthed. In peak periods during the hot summer months the fleet can transport as many as forty thousand people a day to and from the charms of Toronto Island.

TORONTO FIRE DEPARTMENT MARINE FIRE STATION #35 (27): Known officially as Station No. 35, this waterfront facility was built in 1972 as part of the new Metro Toronto Ferry Docks complex. Operating out of No. 35 is the Toronto Fire Department's boat *William Lyon Mackenzie*, named for the city's first mayor who served in 1834, the year Toronto was born. Mackenzie's namesake was launched in 1964 at the Russel Bros. Ltd. shipyard in Owen Sound, Ontario. The *Mackenzie* replaced the obsolete wooden-hulled *Charles A. Reed*, which had seen service on Toronto Bay since 1923 and valiantly fought the tragic *Noronic* blaze in 1949 (see 25). The *William Lyon Mackenzie* is powered by twin Cummins diesels, is 81 feet (24.7 metres) in length, 20 feet (6 metres) wide, and draws 8 feet (2.5 metres) of water. The vessel has a displacement of 110 tons (100 tonnes) and is crewed by a ship's captain and engineer plus a fire captain and two firefighters. Pumps can provide over 7,000 gallons (31,800 litres) of water per minute to four four-inch monitors, three fixed on the wheelhouse and fore and aft decks and one atop the giraffe. This giraffe can attain a maximum height of 54 feet (16.5 metres) and has a full 360-degree swing. The *William Lyon Mackenzie* responds to approximately one hundred calls each year, the most significant to date having involved the inferno aboard the *Orient Trader* in July of 1965. During the winter months, the *Mackenzie* is kept busy breaking ice throughout the harbour. The Marine Unit and the *Mackenzie* will be relocated to the Harbourfront Hall on Queen's Quay West at Maple Leaf Quay when the new facility opens in the summer of 1999.

HARBOUR SQUARE PARK (28): Due west of the Ferry Docks and the Toronto Fire Department's Marine Unit is a small 7.5-acre (3-hectare) city park that grew out of negotiations between Campeau Corporation (the company that built the nearby Harbour Castle Hotel), the Toronto Harbour Commission, and the City of Toronto.

\* \* \* \* \*

BAY STREET: The most likely derivation of this name is rather uninteresting — the thoroughfare ran to or from (depending which way you were headed) Toronto Bay. A less likely, but certainly more entertaining, story suggests that Bay Street actually started off as Bear Street. Legend has it that in the very earliest years of our community's life a bear had been startled while rummaging in the woods near today's City Hall on Queen Street and to escape his pursuers, made for the water by way of a path that has developed into today's Bear, oops, Bay Street.

WATERPARK PLACE (29): The first phase of the Campeau Corporation's impressive WaterPark Place waterfront development at 20 Bay Street opened in December of 1986. Known as Reed Stenhouse Tower after its major tenant, an international insurance brokerage firm, the twenty-six-storey, 486,000-square-foot (45,150-square-metre) office tower is clad in polished, rose-coloured granite and green reflective glass. Immediately to the south is 10 Bay Street, an eighteen-storey, 282,000-square-foot (26,200-square-metre) tower that opened late 1988.

\*   \*   \*   \*   \*

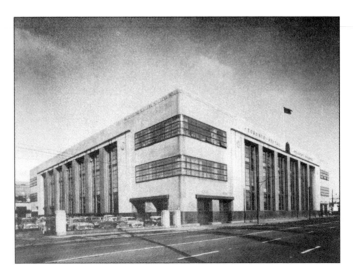

Postal Delivery building, now incorporated into the Air Canada Centre (30). **Courtesy of Canadian Architectural Archives, University of Calgary Library PAN 541132-2**

## Proceed north on Bay Street

AIR CANADA CENTRE (30): Located just a short walk north of Queen's Quay at the Bay Street and Lake Shore Boulevard corner is the $288-million Air Canada Centre, the new home of the Toronto Maple Leafs and Toronto Raptors. Ground was broken on March 12, 1997, and at that time the modern new facility was scheduled to be the home of just the city's National Basketball League team. The Leafs had yet to decide where to build their new arena and were still assessing possible sites that included a location over the Union Station train sheds, a parcel of land northeast of the Yonge Street and Highway 401 cloverleaf, and land at Exhibition Place occupied by the grandstand. In February 1998, management of Maple Leaf Gardens and the Leafs team purchased the Raptors and the Air Canada Centre for $350 million. With the purchase the hockey team finally got its new arena, although obviously major modifications would have to be made to accommodate hockey. It is anticipated that the basketball team will play its 1999 home games in the new Air Canada Centre with the hockey team moving in later that year. If history repeats itself, as it often does, the Maple Leafs will win the Stanley Cup the first season in the new building, just as the team did back in 1931–32 when it played for the first time in the then-brand-new Maple Leaf Gardens. Incidentally, the new structure will incorporate the facade of the former Postal Delivery Building that stood on the site. The construction of this building began in 1938, but was not completed until after the end of the war. Included as part of the facade will be the original sculpted medallions that highlighted the history of communications.

* * * * *

## Return to Queen's Quay and proceed west

510 SPADINA LIGHT RAPID TRANSIT (LRT) LINE: The first section of the new Spadina LRT line opened as the 604 Harbourfront line on June 22, 1990. The cars ran in a tunnel under Bay Street from Union Station to Queen's Quay then via a surface centre-of-the-road reservation on Queen's Quay to a loop at Spadina Avenue. On July 27, 1997, this line was combined with the new 510 Spadina LRT line with service now provided from Union Station to the Spadina station on the Bloor-Danforth subway line. Historically, there had been electric streetcars on both lower Bay Street (from 1927 until 1965) and Spadina Avenue (horsecars in 1878, followed by electric vehicles until 1948). There is talk of constructing a new LRT line along Queen's Quay to Bathurst Street and then on to Exhibition Place.

**33 HARBOUR SQUARE (31):** This 540-unit condominium building opened in 1976 while 55-65 HARBOUR SIDE, with 602 condominium units, opened three years later. Both these Campeau-built structures were to be part of a massive Harbour Castle Hotel-condominium complex, but now, except for the overhead walkway, are not connected in any way.

**TORONTO TRANSPORTATION COMMISSION'S ISLAND FERRY DOCKS (site of, 32):** When the Toronto Transportation Commission took over the operation of the Island ferry service from the privately owned Toronto Ferry Company in April of 1927, the Commission quickly built a new and more modern mainland terminal on this site. It was from here that the eight vessels in the TTC's newly acquired ferry fleet began operating to Ward's Island, Island Park (now Centre Island), and Hanlan's Point. The eight members of the original fleet (and their year of construction) were *Luella* (1880), *John Hanlan* (1884), *Mayflower* (1890), *Primrose* (1890), *Jasmine* (1892), *Clark Bros.* (1901), *Blue Bell* (1906), and *Trillium* (1910). Over the next few years, the TTC acquired a couple of smaller craft, *Aylmer* and *Buttercup*, to carry freight from the city dock to the hundreds of residents and multitude of stores on the Island, and *Mary T*, *Miss York*, and *Miss Simcoe* to provide a highly popular sightseeing service through the Island lagoons. The former fire boat *T.J. Clark* was rebuilt, put into service as a passenger vessel in 1930 and five years later, the newly built *William Inglis* arrived followed in 1939 by the *Sam McBride* and the *Thomas Rennie* eleven years later. In 1962, the TTC turned over Island ferry operations to the Metro Toronto Parks Department (now Toronto Parks), who continued to utilize this facility until the new docks in the Harbour Castle Hotel complex to the east (see 23) were ready in 1972. The 1927 facility was then demolished and no traces of what was one of the happiest (and noisiest) places in Toronto remain.

**TORONTO HARBOUR COMMISSION (THC) BUILDING (33):** It's hard to believe that when the pillared THC building was built some eighty years ago the waters of Toronto Bay lapped at its front steps. The need for a new head office building was recognized soon after the Toronto Harbour Commission was established in 1911. In 1916, a site on the water's edge just east of the foot of Bay Street was selected in order to, as the minute book declares, "demonstrate the Harbour Commissioners' faith in the future of Toronto's waterfront." A year later, the architectural firm of Chapman and McGiffin (Alfred Chapman was also responsible for the Princes' Gates (84) at the Exhibition Grounds as well as many other Toronto landmarks) submitted plans for a handsome building to be constructed of Indiana limestone. Work began almost immediately and by mid-1918, the THC's new $245,000 building was ready for occupancy. Since then, successive waves of landfilling have resulted in the building appearing to have retreated from the harbour's edge. Obviously, the building has stayed in place. The waterfront has changed! Note the unusual, Americanized spelling of the word "Harbor" carved at the top of the building. Today it houses both the offices of the THC as well those of several other businesses.

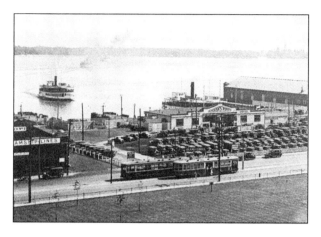

TTC streetcars provide service to the Toronto Island ferry docks near the foot of Bay Street, 1924.

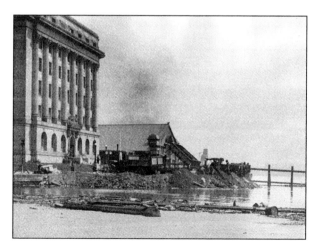

Creating new land south of the Toronto Harbour Commission Building, 1923.

Former WORKMEN'S COMPENSATION BOARD (WCB) BUILDING/ONTARIO PROVINCIAL POLICE HEADQUARTERS (OPP), (34): This building was originally built for the Workmen's (now Workers') Compensation Board (WCB) in 1953. This board was established to administer the Workmen's (Workers') Compensation Act that was passed by the provincial government back in 1915. The act was designed to assist, either financially and/or through retraining, those workers who are injured or get sick as a result of their work. Following the move of the WCB to new premises at 2 Bloor Street East in 1974, the building was acquired by the Ontario Provincial Police and in September of 1975, became the force's general headquarters. One hundred and eighty-nine OPP detachments throughout Ontario reported through sixty district offices to senior staff in this building. In addition, the Special Investigation, Intelligence, and Technical Support branches had offices at 90 Harbour Street. The OPP headquarters were relocated to Orillia, Ontario, over a period of years in the mid-1990s with the new headquarters officially opened on September 16, 1995. Today the building houses a variety of offices.

NUMBER ONE YORK QUAY (35): This 812-unit condominium complex consists of two forty-storey towers and was completed in 1989.

\* \* \* \* \*

Former TORONTO FERRY COMPANY BUILDING, 145 Queen's Quay West (36): The little wooden structure at the foot of York Street is the oldest building on Toronto's ever-changing waterfront. It was originally built in 1907 as part of the Toronto Ferry Company's new docking facility which, prior to landfilling operations, was much further inland over at the foot of Bay Street. The original buildings on the site had been destroyed in a serious fire earlier in the year. When the running of the Island ferry fleet was turned over to the Toronto Transportation Commission twenty years later, a new dock and waiting room were erected south of the newly laid-out Queen's Quay (see 32) and the little building was left without a use. As the waterfront was filled in behind it, the former waiting room was left high and dry. In August of 1927, the Toronto Harbour Commission came to its rescue and the frail little structure was carefully moved to its present location. For the next few years it was used as a storage building. Then, in 1953, the Royal Canadian Yacht Club (RCYC) (see 176) leased it, made renovations, and turned the building into their City Station where club members awaited the RCYC launches running to the Island clubhouse. In 1982, the RCYC moved their City Station to the foot of Parliament Street (see 8). Today, a restaurant, a visitor centre, and a company offering harbour cruises occupy the historic Pier 7 waterfront landmark.

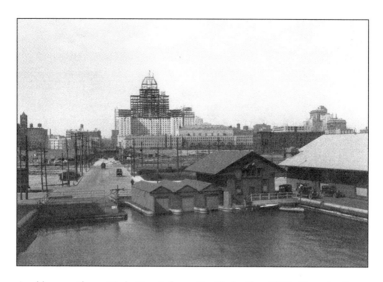

Looking north up York Street from the York slip, 1928. Toronto Ferry Company waiting room (36) at northeast corner of slip. The Royal York Hotel nears completion.

\* \* \* \* \*

YORK STREET: The true derivation of this thoroughfare's name is lost in antiquity. However, if one were to speculate, one plausible reason might be that farmers from west of the Town of York travelling to the St. Lawrence Market (which was, and still is, at the Front and Jarvis corner) might have detoured into town via this still-unnamed street to avoid the quagmire near the Yonge and Queen intersection. Perhaps it was simply the travellers' alternate street into York and was eventually renamed York Street. We do know for certain that the term "York" itself is taken from the title of King George III's second eldest son Frederick, the Duke of York.

\* \* \* \* \*

# Harbourfront Centre (* indicates Harbourfront Centre sites)

The original Harbourfront came into existence in 1972 following the federal government's announcement (co-incident with that year's election campaign) that it would expropriate approximately 80 acres (32 hectares) of property located along the waterfront between York Street on the east and Stadium Road on the west. Included in the expropriation would be a number of industries, some warehouses and factories, railway sidings, wharves and slips, as well as the site of the former, and now demolished, Maple Leaf baseball stadium. It was estimated that the cost of this "gift" would be almost $9 million. While many of the old structures were then demolished, a few others, such as the Terminal Warehouse, an ice plant, and the Direct-Winter's truck depot (now York Quay Centre) were either fully restored or received major renovations. In short order green spaces were developed, several new buildings erected and sidewalks, roadways, and a picturesque 2-mile-long (3.2 kilometres) promenade along the water's edge laid out. These physical changes, combined with an ever-changing programme of year-round events, soon transformed acres of wasteland into one of Toronto's major popular attractions. In 1990 Harbourfront was reconstituted as Harbourfront Centre, a non-profit charitable organization created to organize and present public activities and events on a much-reduced ten-acre site. To best way to describe the multitude of activities and variety of buildings found throughout Harbourfront Centre is to look at them individually. Harbourfront Centre's various information booths can supply additional information. Signs along the way also describe the history of the area.

## * YORK QUAY:

Without question, one of the most beautifully restored buildings in the country, and a restoration rivalling any similar project anywhere on the continent, is the QUEEN'S QUAY TERMINAL (37). It was built over a ten-month period in 1926–1927 at a cost of $3 million by the Toronto Terminal Warehouse Company Limited, who described their new building sitting on 12 1/2 acres (5 hectares) of reclaimed land as "an indispensable link connecting producer, distributor and seller with the customer." Faced with a huge bill to demolish the structure, the developers decided instead to approach the building's future in a different way and spent more than $60 million on its transformation. When constructed in the mid-1920s as a mammoth 1-million-square-foot (92,900-square-metre) warehouse, it was one of the largest buildings in the country and the first to be built of poured concrete. As recently as 1962 the warehouse housed such diverse commodities as paint compounds and pigments, automotive brake parts and batteries, brewers' supplies, and food colourings and flavourings. In room 211 a company started by Woodbridge, Ontario's own Elizabeth Arden warehoused its various fragrances. On the main floor was a branch of the TD Bank and a popular restaurant called the Skipper, an obvious name given the old building's connection with the commercial activities along the waterfront.

Today, Queen's Quay Terminal is home to more than one hundred food stores, specialty shops, and restaurants plus 400,000 square feet (37,160 square metres) of office space and seventy-two luxury condominiums on four newly constructed levels atop the original eight-storey structure. Located on the third floor of Queen's Quay Terminal is the Premier Dance Theatre, the only theatre on the North American continent designed specifically for dance. Located in the former ice-making plant that was built in 1926 to supply ice to the Terminal Warehouse and, for a time, to the Royal York Hotel up on Front Street, is the 450-seat DuMaurier Theatre Centre. Nearby, in a building that formerly housed the generating plant that produced electrical power for the entire Terminal Warehouse complex, is the Power Plant art gallery.

\* YORK QUAY CENTRE (38), located in the former Direct-Winters Transport administration building built in the mid-1940s, is now home to a multitude of performance, dance, and exhibition spaces.

\* South of the York Quay Centre is THE POND which during the winter months is transformed into a the country's largest artificial skating rink.

\* Just west of it is the MOLSON PLACE (39) amphitheatre, which has seating for 1,750 with standing room for thousands more.

\* JOHN QUAY:
John Quay gets its name from the fact that it's at the foot of John Street, a thoroughfare whose name honours John Graves Simcoe, Ontario's first lieutenant-governor and founder of the City of Toronto.

\* Joining the York Quay with the John Quay is the AMSTERDAM BRIDGE (40) erected across the slip in the mid-1970s and named in honour of Toronto's twin city in Holland.

\* On the west side of the bridge is a former warehouse now known as PIER 4 (41). Built by the Toronto Harbour Commission on land reclaimed from Toronto Bay in just seventy-six days in the winter of 1930 the project was a "make work" project undertaken during the early part of the Great Depression. Originally, the 432-foot-long (131.7 metres), sixteen-bay structure was known simply as Transit Shed No. 4. It had an interior storage space of 25,000 square feet (2,323 square metres) and its floors were solid maple.

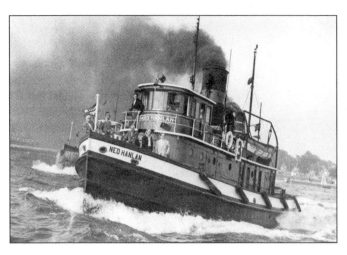

Tug *Ned Hanlan*. Its new home is alongside The Pier (42).

    * Today, the Pier 4 complex includes the Pier 4 Storehouse restaurant and THE PIER (42), Heritage Toronto's updated version of the Marine Museum of the Upper Lakes which was located for many years in the last of the ancient Stanley Barracks buildings in Exhibition Place.

*   *   *   *   *

    * Nearby is a statue of Toronto's world champion sculler Ned Hanlan which was sculpted in 1926 by one of Canada's foremost artists, Emanuel Hahn. This statue originally stood at the west end of the Canadian National Exhibition grounds. It was subsequently moved to a new location in front of the former Marine Museum at the east end of the grounds and in 1998 relocated once again to The Pier at Harbourfront Centre. Interestingly, as Ned had been dead more than fifteen years when the idea of his memorial was finally approved, another champion sculler from Toronto, Joe Wright Jr., helped out as stand-in model. Berthed adjacent to The Pier is the historic tug *Ned Hanlan* which was launched here in Toronto in 1932 and served on Toronto Bay until retired in 1965. Plans call for the tug's eventual restoration and return to use for special cruises on the Bay.

*   *   *   *   *

# Leaving Harbourfront Centre, continue west on Queen's Quay

On the waterfront south of the Radisson Plaza Hotel Admiral (opened 1986) and Admiral Point condominiums (opened 1987) is the TORONTO POLICE DEPARTMENT MARINE UNIT (43). This Crang and Boake-designed building comes complete with a 90-foot (27-metre) lookout tower (with 128 steps), which opened in 1986. The new tower actually replaced a wooden lookout structure that had stood on this same site since 1929. Up until 1982, policing the harbour was the responsibility of the Toronto Harbour Commission's own harbour police. In that year, that organization became part of the city's police department and was designated the Marine Unit. During the sailing season, April 1 to October 31, the men and women of the Marine Unit patrol 27 miles (43.4 kilometres) of waterfront from Marie Curtis Park in Etobicoke on the west to the Rouge River in Scarborough on the east. The actual area patrolled is some 460 square miles (1,191 square kilometres) and runs out to the International Boundary between Canada and the United States in mid-Lake Ontario. The complement of vessels in the Marine Unit fleet consists primarily of fibreglass, aluminum, and welded steel plate craft of various sizes, plus several Zodiacs. In addition there is a trio of unusual vessels including a thirty-three-foot mahogany-planked launch powered by a 350 HP gasoline engine. MU #5 was purchased in 1940 and restored through public funding in 1989. MU #3 is a thirty-four-foot fibreglass Tyler Nelson with superior seaworthiness characteristics for all-weather general patrol, emergency response (it is equipped with fire-fighting capabilities) and long-range search and rescue uses. MU #3 is powered by twin one-hundred-horsepower turbo diesels and equipped with four life rafts allowing a mass rescue of up to three hundred persons. A new addition is MU #6, a twenty-five-foot aluminum air boat for winter operations on ice. The water in the slip adjacent to the boathouse is kept free of ice in the winter months through the use of "bubble guns." With the amalgamation of the Harbour Police with the Metro force in 1982, lifesaving responsibilities were also transferred. Actually, the city's first lifesaving force was a volunteer group that was formed in 1857, becoming a permanent paid force in 1912. Today, the Marine Unit is responsible for eighty lifeguards and their thirty lifeboats, some of which are more than sixty-five-years-old.

\* \* \* \* \*

REES STREET: Born in Bristol, England in 1800, Dr. William Rees came to York (Toronto) in 1829 where he began a medical practice. In 1837 he built a wharf on the south side of Front Street, opposite John Street, where he opened a public bath for the use of immigrants. Next to the wharf, he built himself a small house where he was to live for the rest of his life. Throughout his medical career, Rees constantly advocated various forms of social medicine including free vaccinations for the poor, an orphans' home, an institution for the treatment of alcoholism and a humane society to prevent cruelty to animals. He was responsible for the establishment of the first Provincial Lunatic Asylum in 1841 which was first housed in the old jail at King and Toronto streets prior to being moved into the vacant Parliament Buildings on Front Street West, just steps from his residence. He was appointed as this pioneering institution's first medical superintendent. Soon thereafter, Rees was severely injured by one of the inmates and was forced to retire. He requested a pension and as compensation the government gave him the paltry sum of $1,000, even though the *Dominion Medical Journal* called him "one of the oldest and most respected practitioners in this province." Rees died, alone, in 1874.

ROBERTSON CRESCENT honours John Ross Robertson, Toronto-born businessman and philanthropist. He was the founder of the *Evening Telegram* newspaper (later the *Toronto Telegram*) which first appeared on city streets on April 18, 1876, and quickly became the city's most popular newspaper. The *Telegram* often featured articles on the city's past with special emphasis on its waterfront history. Thus, the naming of a street here on the waterfront is particularly appropriate. With the arrival of another city newspaper, the *Toronto Star* (see 19) in 1892, the stage was set for many fierce newspaper battles, the most famous of which involved 16-year-old Marilyn Bell and the young swimmer's conquest of Lake Ontario (see 109). The *Telegram* ceased publication on Saturday, October 30, 1971. Just two days later, many of the "Tely's" former employees cheered as their new paper, the *Toronto Sun*, made its appearance.

Having lost his daughter to the ravages of scarlet fever, Robertson became deeply involved in the early development of the now-famous Hospital for Sick Children. John Ross Robertson died on May, 31, 1918.

HARBOURFRONT FIRE HALL (proposed site of, 44): As this guide was being written plans were underway to build a new fire hall to serve the fast-growing Harbourfront community. It will be located on the south side of Queen's Quay West and on the east side of the Peter Street slip. It's hoped that a fire museum will eventually be part of this facility.

* * * * *

## Proceed north on Rees Street

Before exploring more of the waterfront and while we're at Rees Street this might be a good place to make a slight detour up Rees, across Lake Shore Boulevard and under the Gardiner Expressway towards SkyDome. Here we'll explore a trio of Toronto landmarks, two new, one old. Let's visit the "old" one first.

The former CANADIAN PACIFIC RAILWAY (CPR) ROUNDHOUSE (45) was erected on this site in 1928–9 as a replacement for an earlier, outmoded facility. This present structure has thirty-two bays accessed by a 120-foot (36.5-metre) diameter turntable. The roundhouse was designed to permit quick servicing and minor repairs to locomotives on the Toronto-Montreal run, thus permitting faster turnaround times on what was a very busy passenger route. Historically, the CPR, which was incorporated in 1881, gained access to the lucrative Toronto market by purchasing smaller, established railway companies like the Credit Valley; the Toronto, Grey, and Bruce; and the Ontario and Quebec; all three of which had running rights into the heart of the city. Eventually, all three of these railways became part of the vast CPR network. When the John Street roundhouse closed in 1986, all of CPR's maintenance operations were moved to the Agincourt Yard in the northeastern part of Toronto. It is hoped that a portion of the roundhouse will eventually become a museum devoted to the history of transportation in Canada. To the east of the historic structure is the newly created Roundhouse Park.

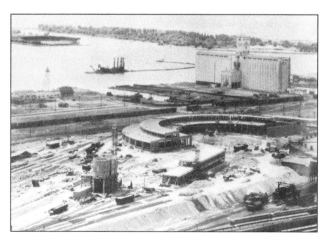

CPR Roundhouse (45) under construction, 1929. Hanlan's Point Stadium (165) at top left.

SKYDOME (46): Next on our tour is the world's first multi-purpose stadium with a fully retractable roof. Work on the massive structure which, it was estimated in mid-1987, would cost $338 million, was financed by both the private and public sectors. The final cost, while well over the estimates, is still somewhat of a secret. Site preparation began in April, 1986, followed by an official ground-breaking ceremony six months later on a rainy October 3. One of the things that had to be done early on in the project was to move the original John Street water pumping station out of the way. It was relocated several hundred feet to the south (see 48) at a cost of close to $18.5 million. This had to be done while ensuring that the station, which was still supplying water to much of downtown Toronto, remained in service.

The "crowning glory" of the new domed stadium is its retractable roof. Covering an area equivalent to a thirty-two-home subdivision and towering 282 feet (86 metres) over the playing field (a thirty-one-storey apartment building could be tucked under the roof, but not without a permit), this engineering marvel is made up of interconnected steel trusses covered with a corrugated steel deck lined with acoustic and thermal insulation and finished outside with white plastic. The roof consists of one fixed-in-place panel plus three additional components each of which is mounted on steel-wheeled bogies riding on steel rails. Two of the moveable panels slide in a north-south direction while a third, semi-circular segment fills the gap by rotating in a half-circle and tucks under the other three panels. When open, one hundred per cent of the field and ninety-one per cent of the seating area is uncovered. At the push of a button the 339,343-square-foot (31,525-square-metre) roof can be opened or closed in just twenty minutes, an activity that has itself become a major attraction in town. SkyDome is home to the Toronto Blue Jays of baseball's American League and the Toronto Argonauts of the Canadian Football League. And the cost of electricity to "cycle" (open and close) the retractable roof? Less than twenty dollars. SkyDome can be configured in several ways, with seating for 54,000 available for baseball games, 56,000 for football, and more than 70,000 for concerts. "The Dome," as it quickly became known, is also the site of numerous consumer and trade shows and a multitude of other events. SkyDome officially opened on a rainy June 3, 1989. In spite of the rain the roof opened on cue and, yes, some guests did get wet. Incidentally, the Jays played in the World Series in SkyDome in both 1992 and 1993, and won on both occasions. The largest crowd thus far has been a 72,000-seat sell-out for the Billy Graham Crusade.

*　*　*　*　*

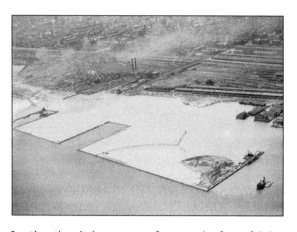

Creating the city's new waterfront at the foot of John Street, 1921. SkyDome would be built on reclaimed land in the centre of this view.

* * * * *

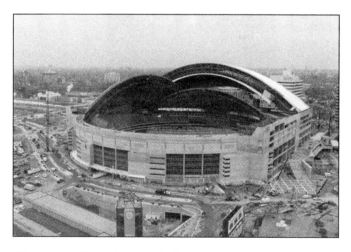

SkyDome (46) nearing completion, 1989. John Street Pumping Station (48) at bottom of view.

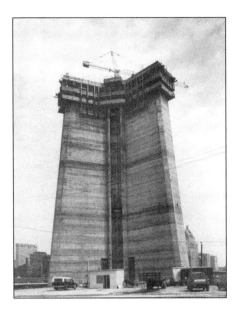

The CN Tower's wooden slip form climbs skyward in this 1973 construction photograph.

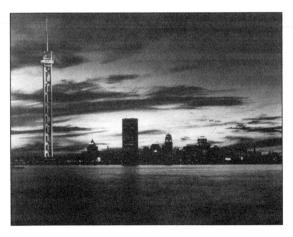

The original CN Tower design called for a three-legged structure.

CN TOWER (47): Here's one structure on Toronto's dazzling waterfront that's certainly not hard to find. Piercing the sky at a dizzying height of 1,815 feet, 5 inches (553.3 metres) work on this, the world's tallest freestanding structure, began in the fall of 1972 when sample borings were made prior to construction of the tower's foundation, which penetrates 50 feet (15 metres) into solid bedrock. Actual above-ground construction commenced on February 6, 1973, followed almost twenty-six months later by the tower's "topping off" when Olga, a huge Sikorsky Skycrane helicopter, lowered the last section of the tower's 365-foot (111-metre) antenna into place. The tower was officially opened on June 26, 1976. The CN Tower was built by Canadian National, one of the world's major transportation, communications, and hospitality enterprises, initially as a communications tower in Metro Centre, a planned redevelopment of the city's long-neglected "railway lands." For various reasons Metro Centre never materialized, but before it was cancelled the tower was under construction. Today, the popular attraction is leased and operated by the TrizecHahn Corp., one of the largest real estate companies in North America. Some features of the CN Tower include six glass-fronted elevators, open and closed observation decks and a four-hundred-seat revolving restaurant at the 1,136 foot (346 metre) level, Sky Pod, the world's highest observation gallery at the 1,465 foot (447 metre) level, a collection of microwave antennas under a flexible doughnut-shaped collar, transmission equipment for sixteen television and FM radio stations as well as all the electrical and mechanical necessities required to keep the tower operating round-the-clock. In May of 1998, a $26-million expansion and revitalization program saw the addition of a new Imax theatre called the Maple Leaf Cinema, two new motion simulator rides, a themed arcade, additional retail spaces — including a duty-free shop (the first in downtown Toronto) — and an interactive display depicting the story behind the building of the CN Tower. By the way, you might be interested in knowing that the tower was built at a cost of $63 million (1976 Canadian dollars), or $2,891.90 an inch.

\* \* \* \* \*

JOHN STREET PUMPING STATION (48), which we pass on the right on our way back down to Queen's Quay, supplies the thirsty city with more than 200 million gallons (909 million litres) of water from Lake Ontario every day. As the original John Street pumping facility was located where the playing field at SkyDome was to be laid out it became necessary to relocate the station some 325 feet (100 metres) to the south at a cost of $18.5 million. Historically, the first company to supply water to Torontonians came into existence in 1841 and was privately owned. Its pumping station was located a few hundred feet north of the present pumping station and served the needs of the eighteen thousand citizens living in a city that was still just seven years old. After thirty years of less-than-satisfactory service, the City of Toronto purchased the company and quickly upgraded all components of the water pumping complex. Over the years, as more and more potable water became necessary, the plant underwent continual expansion and when plans were announced to build SkyDome work began on relocating the facility to its present location south of the Dome. Water from the station is directed to several large reservoirs located around the city from which distribution takes place to the city's thousands of industrial, commercial, and residential users. Incidentally, the tall concrete structure houses a huge surge tank positioned in such a way so as to prevent the rupturing of pipes due to air pressure buildup should pump failure occur. In effect, it's a "burp tank."

## Return to Queen's Quay and proceed west

THE RIVIERA ON QUEEN'S QUAY (49): At the northwest corner of Rees Street and Queen's Quay is one of the many new condominium towers being built along the city's waterfront to take advantage of the both the view and the proximity to the heart of Toronto. This 342-unit condominium is expected to be ready for occupancy in September, 1999.

Returning to the south side of Lake Shore Boulevard we enter MAPLE LEAF QUAY. This part of Harbourfront Centre was named for Maple Leaf Mills Limited, a busy waterfront industry whose office and laboratory buildings and two two-million bushel grain elevators occupied this site for years. The elevators were demolished in 1983 after the company moved from Toronto, consolidating operations in Windsor, Ontario.

On the east side of the Quay, and adjacent to the Rees Street slip, is the NAUTICAL CENTRE (50) where students can learn all the intricacies of being safe and responsible boaters.

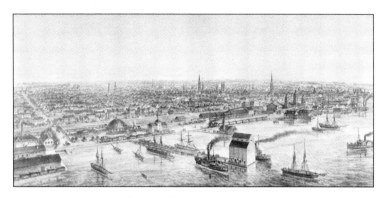

Toronto's waterfront at the foot of Brock Street (now Spadina Avenue) was a hive of activity in 1876.

HARBOURFRONT ANTIQUE MARKET (51), located on the north side of Queen's Quay, is one of the most popular attractions along this part of Toronto's busy waterfront.

One door west, at the northeast corner of Queen's Quay and Spadina Avenue, is the former head office building of MAPLE LEAF MILLS LIMITED.

510 SPADINA LIGHT RAIL TRANSIT (LRT) LINE: This LRT route ("light rail transit" is simply a modern term for the old-fashioned word "streetcar") was opened with appropriate ceremonies on July 27, 1997. It was combined with the 604 Harbourfront route, which had opened seven years earlier, to provide service from Union Station via Bay Street (underground), Queen's Quay, and Spadina Avenue to an underground connection with the Bloor-Danforth subway at the Spadina station. While the line is new, in actual fact, streetcars on Spadina Avenue are not new. Starting as far back as 1878 horsedrawn streetcars operated on Spadina. A new route called Belt Line (operating via Spadina Avenue, Bloor, Sherbourne, and King streets) was introduced in 1891 and the route electrified the following year. In 1923 the Spadina route was reinstated and double-end vehicles (with trolley poles at both ends of the car and seats that flipped over at the end of the line) were introduced. The Spadina line continued to operate until 1948 when shortages of electricity forced the replacement of the electric vehicles with gas buses. While new sources of electricity were eventually developed, the buses remained. Nearly a half-century later electric streetcars returned to Spadina Avenue.

LOWER SPADINA AVENUE: The original Spadina Avenue was laid out in the late 1820s by William Warren Baldwin, who, as a young man of 24, had arrived with the rest of the Baldwin family in York (Toronto) in 1799. Baldwin was an extremely accomplished gentleman being a medical doctor, lawyer, architect, and successful politician. In 1818, he built for himself a house on the escarpment overlooking the young town, a house he called Spadina (correctly pronounced Spad-eena) after the Mississauga Indian word for "a sudden rise of land." Spadina Avenue was laid out as a grand thoroughfare two chains wide (132 feet, 40.2 metres) cut through the forest and leading to Baldwin's home on the hill from Lot, now Queen Street, to the south. The house burned in 1835 and a newer (1868) Spadina House now occupies the site. It's located just to the east of Casa Loma, "the castle on the hill." Up until 1884, the section of today's Spadina Avenue from Queen Street to Front Street was called Brock Street in tribute to James Brock, a former land owner and the cousin of Major-General Sir Isaac Brock, the hero of the War of 1812 who helped repel the American invaders at Queenston Heights and was killed in the battle. The bridge over the railway tracks that connects Front Street with today's Lake Shore Boulevard replaced an old narrow steel bridge that was erected in 1925–1926 and had badly deteriorated as a result of years of being drenched with hot smoke from the hundreds of steam engines that passed under it daily.

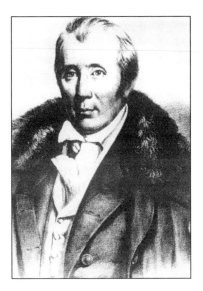

Dr. William Warren Baldwin, the "architect" of Spadina Avenue.

## Spadina Quay:

The land to the west of Lower Spadina Avenue was reclaimed from Toronto Bay in the mid-1910s and almost before the land had dried the DOMINION SHIPBUILDING COMPANY (site of, 52) had moved onto the property and soon began turning out much needed freighters, at the rate of one a month, for the war effort. Following the end of the so-called "war to end all wars" the Hamilton Bridge company occupied the site until once again war broke out. This time however, warships were of paramount importance and the newly formed Dufferin Shipbuilding Company bought out Hamilton Bridge and quickly began turning out 225-foot-long (68.6 metres) minesweepers for Atlantic convoy duty. Dufferin and its successors, Toronto Shipbuilding and Redfern Construction, built a total of fifty-six minesweepers, ten of the "Bangor" class for the Royal Canadian Navy and forty-six "Algerine" class for the Royal Navy. Shipyards similar to this one helped make Canada the third largest shipbuilding nation in the world during the war years. Following the end of hostilities, Dufferin Shipbuilding's administration building, erected in 1939, was acquired by the American Trucking Association.

\*   \*   \*   \*   \*

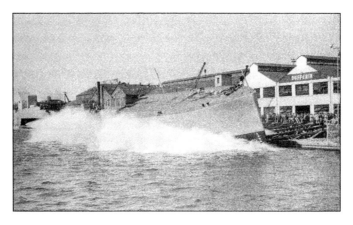

Another minesweeper hits the water at the shipbuilding yard (52) at the foot of Spadina Avenue, 1944.

Now sitting on the north side of this historic shipyard site (the 1986 extension of Queen's Quay westerly from Spadina to Stadium Road bisected the yard) is the spectacular KING'S LANDING (53) condominium/office complex that was designed by Arthur Erickson. Erickson is also responsible for the spectacular Roy Thompson Hall, Toronto's premier music auditorium, on King Street West.

On the south side of Queen's Quay and just west of the foot of Spadina Avenue is SPADINA QUAY PARKLANDS (54) in which a pike-spawning habitat and wetlands are being developed. The latter's creation (the first wetlands on the north side of the harbour in many, many decades) will encourage pike to enter and spawn.

Adjacent to the park is the SPADINA MARINA (55) with mooring facilities for approximately 120 vessels. This marina is open to the public and affords a magnificent place for boat owners, and those who wish they could be boat owners, to mingle. A three-level parking garage for 340 cars sits under Spadina Marina.

THE MUSIC GARDEN (56), a new, privately funded addition to the Harbourfront Park system, was conceived by internationally renowned cellist Yo Yo Ma and garden designer Julie Moir Messervy. It was originally destined for the City of Boston's waterfront, but when that proposal failed the pair approached Toronto officials who warmly welcomed the idea. The concept for the park is based on J.S. Bach's Cello Suite No. 1 as interpreted by Yo Yo Ma. Each dance movement of the suite is reflected in the park's elaborate design: the Prelude by an undulating riverscape; Allemande by a forest grove of wandering trails; Courante by a swirling path through a wildflower meadow; Sarabande by a conifer grove; Menuett by a formal flower parterre; and Gigue by giant grass steps.

FIVE HUNDRED QUEEN'S QUAY WEST (57), a new 181-unit (plus penthouses) condominium development, is scheduled for completion late in 1998 and is located, thankfully, on the north side of the street.

LOWER PORTLAND STREET: The original Portland Street, north of Lake Shore Boulevard and the railway tracks, was named for William Henry Cavendish Bentinck, the Third Duke of Portland, prime minister of England in 1807, fourteen years after the community was established by Simcoe. This portion of the street is newly laid out.

\* \* \* \* \*

Just west of the Lower Portland Street corner, and still on the north side of Queen's Quay, is QUEEN'S HARBOUR (58), a 276-unit condominium project scheduled for occupancy in March, 1999.

Returning to the south side of Queen's Quay we see the former CANADA MALTING COMPANY complex (site of 59). Established in 1900, the Canada Malting Company moved to this property, reclaimed from Toronto Bay by the Toronto Harbour Commission, in 1928 and spent $700,000 erecting a number of buildings and storage silos. The company soon began processing barley and other ingredients into malt for various breweries and distilleries as well as for food processors and a variety of pharmaceutical manufacturers. On several occasions increasing business forced the company to expand the plant. With the company's abandonment of the site in late 1987 a search began to find a suitable reuse of the buildings and silos. In late 1997, the Metronome Canada Foundation announced a fundraising campaign to convert the complex into a one-of-a-kind centre to celebrate all facets of the Canadian music industry. Included in the $70-million concept will be an eight-hundred-seat theatre, a music business centre, a digital development centre and a Canadian Music Hall of Fame, the latter in the 1928 silos.

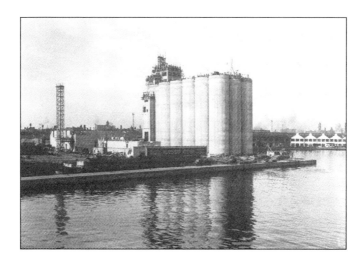

Work continues on the new Canada Malting elevator near the foot of Bathurst Street, 1926.

THE WATERFRONT SCHOOL (60), which serves the fast-growing waterfront community, opened its doors in September, 1997, and offers classes kindergarten through grade eight. Incorporated in the modern building is the Harbourfront Community Centre.

BATHURST STREET: Until 1931, Bathurst Street, which was named in 1820 for Henry, third Earl of Bathurst, the British Secretary of War and the Colonies from 1812–1827, only ran as far south as Front Street where traffic was forced to veer southwest over a large, steel bridge across the railway tracks and proceed west, north of Fort York, on Garrison Road to the latter thoroughfare's intersection with Strachan Avenue. In 1931, the bridge seen in the distance was pivoted to come into a north-south axis and a new roadbed built to connect with the recently opened Lake Shore Boulevard to the south. Incidentally, that bridge was originally built at the western approach to the city to carry trains over the mouth of the Humber River. It was erected there in 1903 by the Grand Trunk Railway (now Canadian National Railways) and when, in 1916, it became too light for the new and heavier steam engines to cross safely was moved to its present location. The reason for its reuse? To save the taxpayers money!

## (Optional) Proceed south on Bathurst Street

TORONTO CITY CENTRE (formerly Toronto Island) AIRPORT MAINLAND DOCK (61): Located at the foot of Bathurst Street, it is from this point that the ferry Maple City (and, when required, Windmill Point) depart on their two-minute run to the airport on the south side of the Western Gap.

TUNNEL TO TORONTO ISLAND (site of, 62): For more than one hundred years there has been talk of building a vehicle bridge or tunnel to connect the mainland with Toronto Island. In fact, a start was made in 1935 on a $1-million, 2000-foot-long (610 metres) vehicular tunnel under the Western Gap. The project was part of Conservative Prime Minister R.B. Bennett's master plan for a number of public works projects all across Canada designed to get Canadians back to work following years of depression. The federal government in Ottawa changed hands soon after work on the tunnel began and although the city fathers screamed they were being victimized by the new prime minister, William Lyon Mackenzie King, the government ordered the tunnel plan shelved. The hole was filled in and that was that. But wait, plans have once again surfaced to provide vehicular access to the airport, only this time it'll be via a bridge over the Western Gap. The first scheme to get vehicles to the Island also involved a bridge, and that was in 1886. So don't hold your breath. There are great views of the city's skyline from this vantage point.

LITTLE NORWAY (site of, 63): Following the invasion of Norway by Germany on April 9, 1940, an attempt was made to establish an air force training camp in France. When this failed, negotiations with the Canadian government began and soon a site in Toronto at the foot of Bathurst Street across the Western Gap from the recently opened Port George VI Island Airport (see 167) was offered. On August 20, 1940, 120 young Norwegian airmen arrived in our city and by September, flight refresher courses using Fairchild trainers, Curtis fighters, Douglas bombers, and Northrop patrol craft were underway at the Island Airport. Soon a busy camp of seventeen buildings with a "population" of one thousand proud Norwegians sprang up across the Gap on the mainland, directly south of the Maple Leaf ball stadium (see 65). Access to and from the airport was via a small cable ferry. Little Norway quickly outgrew its Toronto facilities and in the spring of 1942, officers, men, and aircraft moved to the Dominion Airport near Gravenhurst in Muskoka. In the spring of 1945, the entire operation was moved to Devon in England.

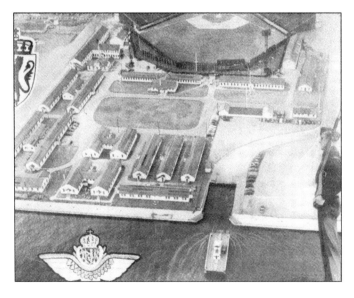

The Little Norway encampment (63) in the early years of the Second World War. Maple Leaf Stadium (65) at top, Western Gap at bottom.

## Return to Queen's Quay

NORWAY PARK (64), at the southwest corner of Queen's Quay and Bathurst Street, was so named to commemorate the presence of the Norwegian air-training base. Under the trio of flagpoles at the north end of the park that fly the Toronto, Canadian, and Norwegian flags, is a boulder transported from Lista in Norway and on which is affixed a special commemorative plaque unveiled by Crown Prince Harald of Norway in 1976. Surrounding the park are the Harbourside, Arcadia, and Windward co-operative housing units. On Stadium Road and Lake Shore Boulevard are special, geared-to-income rental units developed by the City of Toronto's Municipal Non-Profit Housing Corporation, Cityhome. At the foot of Stadium Road and at the southwest corner of Queen's Quay and Bathurst Streets are two 250-unit senior citizen condominiums called The Harbours. Eventually, the Bathurst Quay community will be home to more than one thousand residents. One of the new streets on the site of the old baseball stadium is Bishop Tutu Boulevard, named out of respect for this Nobel Peace Prize winner who visited Toronto two years after he won the award in 1984. At the northwest corner of the Bathurst Street and Queen's Quay intersection is another new condominium development. Plans call for The Atrium on Queen's Quay, a 298-unit project, to be ready for occupancy in late 1999.

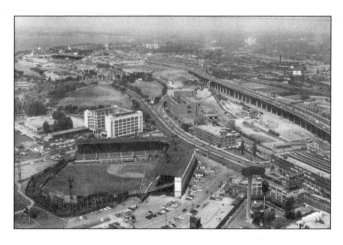

Maple Leaf Stadium (65), Tip Top Tailors (74), Molson Breweries (70), Fort York (81), and CFMT Studios (66) are seen in this early 1960s view.

# Proceed north on Bathurst Street

MAPLE LEAF STADIUM (site of, 65): Toronto got its first professional baseball team in 1885. In the ensuing years the team played at numerous parks all over the city including a major facility at the Island (see 165). In 1926, Lol Solman, who owned both the ball team and the ferry boats that fans used to get to the Island stadium, had a disagreement with the city fathers over the operation of his ferry fleet. The city expropriated his Toronto Ferry Company and in retaliation, Solman leased land from the Toronto Harbour Commission and moved his International League ball team to a new stadium on land at the southwest corner of today's Lake Shore Boulevard and Bathurst Street intersection. On a rainy April 29, 1926 the Toronto Maple Leaf baseball team won their opening game at the new stadium, defeating the Reading Keystones 6–5. That same year, the team went on to win the Little World Series Championship. Over the next four decades, the Leafs won five International League pennants and four Governor's Cup Championships at the stadium. During the period 1951 to 1960, the team was owned by flamboyant Hamilton, Ontario-born Jack Kent Cooke, a former encyclopedia salesman. Cooke eventually sold the team and moved to the United States where he purchased the Los Angeles Kings National Hockey League team and Los Angeles Lakers basketball team and built that city's Forum. Cooke later owned the Washington Redskins of the National Football League. Interestingly, it was Jack Kent Cooke who tried to bring major league baseball to Toronto as early as 1960, but he was stymied by the politicians of the day. As the years went by interest in the International League Maple Leaf baseball team began to wane and on September 4, 1967, only 802 stalwart fans were on hand to see the Leafs play their final game, a 7–2 loss to the Syracuse Chiefs. Maple Leaf Stadium, where Torontonians saw their first ever Sunday baseball game on May 7, 1950, was demolished in 1968. A little more Toronto trivia, some former Maple Leafs players, managers, and coaches who made it to the major leagues: Sparky Anderson, Ed Barrow, Rico Carty, Al Cicotte, Chuck Dressen, Burleigh Grimes, Carl Hubbell, Sparky Lyle, Mel McGaha, Bubba Morton, Pat Scantlebury, Luke Sewell, Reggie Smith, Ozzie Virgil, and Dick Williams.

\* \* \* \* \*

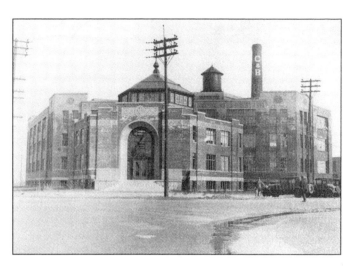

Crosse and Blackwell, now CFMT Studios at the Bathurst Street-Lake Shore boulevard intersection, 1928.

CFMT STUDIOS (66): At the southeast corner of Bathurst and Lake Shore Boulevard West are the studios of Toronto's multicultural television station CFMT, Channel 47. This station went on the air in 1979 and broadcasts programs in numerous languages that reflect most of the ethnic cultures living in the Greater Toronto area. The building CFMT now occupies was originally built for $500,000 in 1927 for Crosse and Blackwell, the famous British jam, pickle, and condiment manufacturers. The original "C&B" company logo can still be seen above the door of this unique "art deco" building designed by the talented Toronto architect Alfred Chapman who was also responsible for such city landmarks as the CNE's Princes' Gates (see 84) and the Toronto Harbour Commission Building (see 33). In 1949, Loblaws, acquired the building as its head office and in 1975 the historic structure was expropriated as part of the Harbourfront project.

\* \* \* \* \*

LAKE SHORE BOULEVARD: Just one year after the passing of the Toronto Harbour Commission Act in 1911, the newly appointed Toronto Harbour Commissioners unveiled their $19-million-dollar (1912 dollars) plan for the redevelopment of the city's long-neglected waterfront. This plan, the creation of the commission's extremely competent chief engineer, Edward Lancelot Cousins (1883–1961), was based, in part, on the Burnham Plan of 1909 for Chicago's waterfront and had as one component the concept of a scenic boulevard along the shore of Lake Ontario with the western section built on land reclaimed from the old Humber Bay. This thoroughfare was to parallel the western lakefront, cross over the Western Gap via a bridge, wind through the Islands, and cross the Eastern Gap on a bridge high enough for the largest ships on the Great Lakes to pass under. Work commenced on the 50-foot-wide (15 metres) Boulevard Drive following the end of the Great War and opened as far as Dowling Avenue in late 1921. The grand scheme for this grand trafficway never fully materialized. In fact, the Boulevard originally ended at Bathurst Street with the continuation to the east known at first as Fleet Street. It wasn't until 1960 that the cross-waterfront traffic artery became known as Lake Shore Boulevard from one end to the other.

\* \* \* \* \*

Former LOBLAWS WAREHOUSE (67): Across the street, on the north side of Lake Shore Boulevard, stands the former warehouse and head office of the prominent Canadian food retailer, Loblaws. This massive structure, which was built in 1927 at a cost of approximately $700,000, has 350,000 square feet (32,515 square metres) of floor space. In addition to warehousing, there were administration offices as well as equipment (in what was described at the time as the most up-to-date grocery warehouse on the continent) for the manufacture and packaging of special Loblaws brands of coffee, tea, cookies, candies, dairy products, and many other items. There was also a large meat department where whole sides of beef arrived by rail to be stored in huge on-site freezers prior to preparation for retail sale in the numerous Loblaw Groceterias around the province. Loblaws was established by Alliston, Ontario-born Theodore Pringle Loblaw who, in 1889 at the age of 17, arrived penniless in Toronto. He obtained a job in a small grocery store operated by a Mr. Cork. Through hard work, he and Cork's son Milton soon opened their own store which by 1910 had grown into a chain of ten one-man grocery stores with the name T.P. Loblaw over the door. Nine years later, Loblaw sold all the stores to an organization called Dominion Stores. Loblaw and Cork then started over and opened Canada's first self-serve, cash-and-carry "groceteria" (as Loblaw himself named it). Today, Loblaws has become one of the world's great food supermarket operations and is now owned by George Weston Limited, another company created by an enterprising Torontonian. All of the operations formerly conducted in the old warehouse building on the corner are now carried out at the company's sprawling Mississauga, Ontario premises.

\* \* \* \* \*

OLD WESTERN GAP (site of, 68): For hundreds of years, the stretch of water separating the west end of the peninsula (after 1858, the Island) from the mainland was located just north of the present Bathurst Street and Lake Shore Boulevard intersection. The approach to Toronto Harbour through this Gap was very dangerous with numerous vessels coming to grief on the rocky shoals just outside the entrance to the Gap. In 1861, a lighthouse was erected on the Queen's Wharf as an aid to navigation through this dangerous entrance to Toronto Bay (see 75). A particularly tragic incident took place one stormy night in late November, 1906, when the steam barge *Resolute*, after failing to gain access to the sheltered waters of the harbour through the Eastern Gap, made her way around the south side of the Island and, finding the depth of water in the Western Gap too little for the coal-laden vessel, was moored off Hanlan's Point until the storm abated. Unfortunately, the winds changed direction and began to batter the little ship unmercifully. The crew decided to make a run for the Eastern Gap, but again, with no luck. Soon the *Resolute* began to sink as she waited out the storm off the Western Gap. Two lifeboats were launched, but as the crew scrambled aboard one of the boats capsized throwing five of the crew into the foaming waters where they drowned. A sixth was washed away from the *Resolute* and he too was lost. As a result of an unsafe Western Gap, six men were drowned. Less than a year later, the Federal Department of Public Works approved the creation of a deeper and safer Western Gap 1,300 feet (396 metres) to the south of the old Gap. This new entrance was ready for the 1911 navigation season. Six years later, as part of the preliminary work on Boulevard Drive, the old Western Gap was filled in.

* * * * *

## Proceed west on the south side of Lake Shore Boulevard

IMPERIAL OIL GAS STATION (69): Imperial Oil Limited, a company established in 1880 in London, Ontario by a group of influential businessmen, purchased a small parcel of land at the southwest corner of Bathurst Street and Lake Shore Boulevard in 1925 and shortly thereafter erected a small service station on the site. Although the station and facilities have been greatly modernized over the years, Imperial still serves gasoline from this corner. Some more Toronto motoring trivia: in the year that Lake Shore Boulevard and Bathurst Street station opened, there were some 304,000 cars in all of Ontario. Today, there are well over a million cars in the Toronto area alone. And, if you had driven up to that Imperial Oil station's pump for some gas in 1925, you would have paid 28.8 cents ... a gallon!

TORONTO'S STREETCARS: Gliding along Fleet Street (as well as Queen's Quay and up and down Bathurst Street and Spadina Avenue) are some of Toronto's fleet of 248 modern electric streetcars. Streetcars have been a part of Toronto since 1861 when the first horsedrawn cars trotted down Yonge Street from the first of Toronto's numerous suburbs, Yorkville, just north of Bloor Street, to the city's business and social centre near King and Jarvis streets. The number of streetcar routes expanded rapidly so that by the time new electric vehicles were introduced in 1892, 19 million passengers were being carried in cars owned by a private company on fifteen different routes over 80 miles (129 kilometres) of track paying an adult fare of five cents cash or twenty-five tickets for one dollar; kids, three cents cash. (Incidentally, it was at this time that the free transfer came into being, a feature still maintained by the present operator.) On September 1, 1921, the municipality-operated Toronto Transportation Commission took over virtually all public transportation responsibilities in the Greater Toronto community of 603,900 citizens. That portion of transit service provided by streetcars continued to expand so that by 1953, there were almost 1,100 of these electrically powered vehicles operating a total of thirty million miles each year over twenty-two routes scattered throughout the city. With the opening of the Yonge subway on March 30, 1954, many streetcar routes were abandoned and more routes were curtailed when the University and Bloor-Danforth subway lines opened in 1963 and 1966 respectively. At one point, the TTC nearly abandoned the streetcar totally, but thanks to a committee of interested citizens, all five TTC commissioners, several of the commission's senior staff and a few far-sighted politicians, the TTC continues to operate streetcars. The first of the Canadian Light Rail Vehicles (CLRV), similar to those seen on Queen's Quay and Spadina Avenue, went into service in 1979 while the larger Articulated Light Rail Vehicles (ALRV) appeared in 1988. Because 511 Bathurst is one of the busiest streetcar routes in the city ALRVs have been assigned to this line. And here's some real Toronto trivia: CLRVs 4000–4005 were prototype cars built in Switzerland while CLRVs 4010–4199 were built in Thunder Bay, Ontario. Incidentally, Toronto streetcars, including a pair of 1951-vintage Presidents' Conference Committee Streamliners numbered 4500 and 4549, are available for private charter by calling the TTC.

FLEET STREET: Just north of Lake Shore Boulevard is Fleet Street, which was created in the early 1920s on land reclaimed by the Toronto Harbour Commission. The thoroughfare was named for the famous London, England, street that, in turn, was named for the River Fleet which it followed. Toronto's Fleet Street originally ran from Strachan Avenue east to Parliament Street. In 1960 most of that thoroughfare was renamed Lake Shore Boulevard with only the present Fleet Street retaining its original name.

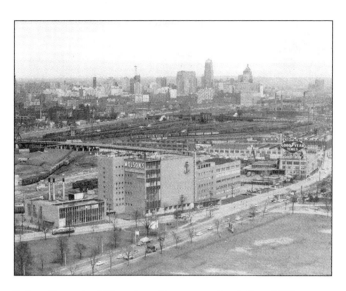

Molson Breweries (70) and a rather sparce city skyline, 1958.

Former MOLSON ONTARIO BREWERIES LIMITED plant (70): The idea of drinking beer is more than 3,500 years old. In fact, research indicates that it was prehistoric man that first enjoyed a "nice cold one." More recently, in 1783 to be exact, eighty-four years before the provinces of Upper and Lower Canada, Nova Scotia, and New Brunswick joined together to form the Dominion of Canada, a young John Molson arrived in Montreal, Quebec, from Lincolnshire, England. Molson joined a fellow immigrant, Thomas Laid, and together they operated a small brewery on the north shore of the St. Lawrence River just outside the city's walled boundary. Two years later, Molson purchased the brewery from Laid, returned to England to settle his estate and, returning to Montreal in July of 1786, began brewing the first few hogsheads of the now famous Molson ale and beer. Today, Molson's is the oldest operating brewery in North America. For its first 169 years of business life the company operated breweries only in the province of Quebec. Then in 1953, Molson's purchased a 10-acre (4-hectare) parcel of land on the north side of Fleet Street just west of Bathurst as the site for its first brewery outside Quebec. Rumour has it that the property was actually purchased from an unsuspecting E.P. Taylor, owner of several competing brewing companies who went ballistic when he learned who had purchased the land. In 1955, the new Molson brewery, described as being the most modern in the world, began producing its first product, Crown and Anchor beer, the company's first ever lager. Over the years the waterfront plant produced several different Molson brands from raw materials that include water, barley malt, cereal grains, and hops. Of special interest is the fact that several brands brewed at the Toronto plant were exported to forty-five of the fifty American states, including Alaska and Hawaii. For business reasons all brewing operations at the Fleet Street plant were transferred to the Etobicoke plant. This plant was then closed, and although the property has been rezoned for residential purposes, at present (1998) there are no plans for redevelopment.

STADIUM ROAD: So named for the nearby Maple Leaf Stadium where the International League baseball Leaf team played from 1926 until 1967. The stadium was demolished in 1968.

\* \* \* \* \*

## (Optional) Proceed south on Stadium Road

NATIONAL YACHT CLUB, 1 Stadium Road (71): The National Yacht Club (NYC) had as its genesis the National Yacht and Skiff Club which was established in 1894 in a former Royal Canadian Yacht Club building which had been moved from the foot of York Street to the foot of Bathurst Street adjacent to the old Queen's Wharf. In 1903, this site was expropriated by the street railway company and the old building was moved again, this time to the northeast corner of what with landfilling has become the Lake Shore Boulevard-Bathurst Street intersection. Back then of course, the site was still on the water's edge. In 1919 the club moved to a new site on what became known as Stadium Road following the construction of the Maple Leaf ball stadium (see 65). Ongoing redevelopment of the waterfront resulted in the club relocating once again, this time onto reclaimed land closer to the Western Gap.

ALEXANDRA YACHT CLUB, 2 Stadium Road (72): Established in 1907, the Alexandra Yacht Club's (AYC) first clubhouse was at the east end of Toronto Bay on Fisherman's Road in an area that was to become the Eastern Harbour Terminals under the newly created Toronto Harbour Commission's grand plan of 1912. The implementation of the plan forced the club to move to the end of a pier jutting into Toronto Bay at Ward's Island at the east end of Toronto Island. After just three years at the Ward's Island location, the clubhouse was totally destroyed in a violent midwinter storm that hit Toronto on January 10, 1919. Club officials then decided to move operations to the protection of a new "Aquatic Reservation" created by the Harbour Commission on the mainland side of the Bay just west of Bathurst Street. With the redevelopment of property fronting on the new

Stadium Road, the AYC moved once again, this time to a new location on reclaimed adjacent to the Western Gap and next door to the National Yacht Club. The present AYC fleet comprises almost one hundred vessels.

A proposal has been submitted to erect a new six-hundred-unit condominium development appropriately named THE YACHT CLUB (73) on property just north of these two clubs. It is scheduled to be ready for occupancy in late 1999.

TIP TOP TAILORS, 637 Lake Shore Boulevard West (74): This handsome, $500,000, five-storey structure was erected in 1929 (a sixth floor was added in 1951) as a men's made-to-order clothing factory by Tip Top Tailors Limited where up to ten thousand suits and overcoats were produced weekly. The steel and concrete building, containing 210,000 square feet (19,500 square metres) of floor space, was built on 3 1/2 acres of land reclaimed by the Toronto Harbour Commission during the massive waterfront redevelopment project approved by City Council in 1912. Tip Top Tailors was established in 1909 by David Dunkleman, a young Polish immigrant who first settled in the United States, then moved to Toronto where he worked for his father, Elias, who was employed as a sub-contractor making buttonholes for local clothing manufacturers. Young David lasted only a short time working for his father and soon opened his own wholesale suit company, but did not do well. He then decided to "go retail" and opened his first store at 245 Yonge Street to the public on March 4, 1911. Needing a name for the new business, David devised a contest that

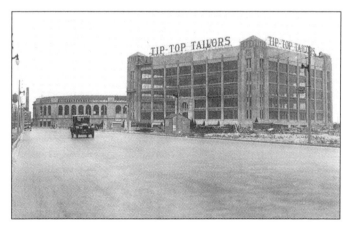

Maple Leaf Stadium (65) and Tip Top Tailors (74) line the south side of an almost car-free Fleet Street (now Lake Shore Blvd. W.), 1929.

would see twenty-five dollars awarded to the person submitting the catchiest name for his new enterprise. When "Tip Top Tailors" was suggested by a local journalist, Dunkleman approved. Tip Top Tailors it would be. During the Second World War, hundreds of thousands of uniforms for Canadian servicemen and women were manufactured in this building. Tip Top Tailors is part of the huge Dylex Diversified organization. ("Dylex" is said to be an acronym for "Damn Your Lousy Excuses," a favourite expression of one of the company founders.) Under the Dylex umbrella are Tip Top, Thrifty's, Biway, and Fairweather.

THE QUEEN'S WHARF LIGHTHOUSE (75): When originally constructed in 1861 this little lighthouse, now on the north side of Lake Shore Boulevard, sat at the end of the Queen's Wharf that jutted into the old West Gap approximately where the car dealership is now located at the Bathurst and Lake Shore intersection. It's estimated that the lighthouse guided more than 300,000 ships of all sizes through the Gap during its half-century of service. In 1911, following several serious accidents that occurred in the Gap, it was decided to build a more easily navigatable and therefore safer Western Gap some 1,300 feet (396 metres) further south. As a result the old lighthouse was left "high and dry." In 1929, the structure was donated by the Toronto Harbour Commission to the city and relocated to its present site in November of that year. The move, from the northwest corner of today's Bathurst and Fleet streets location to the streetcar loop in front of the former Molson's plant, was accomplished using wooden rollers and real horse power. The historic relic is now under the care of Heritage Toronto.

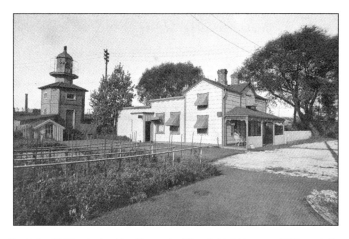

In this 1928 photo the Queen's Wharf Lighthouse (75) and the lighthouse keeper's residence on a site now occupied by a car dealership at the northwest corner of Bathurst St. and Lake Shore Blvd. W.

HMCS YORK (76): South of Lake Shore Boulevard is the Naval Reserve Unit HMCS York whose predecessor was the Toronto Half Company that was formed in 1923 and met for a time in the Navy League Building at 1395 Lake Shore Boulevard West (see 113). In 1941, the unit was commissioned HMCS York to commemorate the British "Exeter" class cruiser HMS *York* that had just been sunk in the Mediterranean Sea by enemy aircraft on May 29, 1941. HMCS York moved into this building in 1946 after a short wartime stint in the HMCS "Auto Building" on the Exhibition Grounds (see 85).

FORT YORK ARMOURY, 660 Fleet Street (77): To the north of Lake Shore Boulevard is Fort York Armoury. Prior to its opening in January, 1935, many Toronto militia units were forced to parade in makeshift drill halls located in hospitals, postal stations, and the like scattered all over the city. To be sure several of the Toronto militia units were able to take advantage of the huge University Avenue Armoury downtown. Finally, the commanding officers of several units that weren't so fortunate approached the federal government to request a new facility for five local militia units, the Royal Regiment of Canada (established in 1862), the Queen's York Rangers (1866), the Corps of Royal Canadian Engineers (1901), the Irish Regiment (1915), and the Toronto Scottish Regiment (1920). The government's answer was the imposing Fort York Armoury which was designed by the local architectural firm of Marani, Lawson, and Morris and built at a cost of $350,000. Interestingly, F.H. Marani was also commanding officer of the Royal Regiment. The insignia of four of the original units, and the mottos of two, can still be seen across the top of the imposing structure

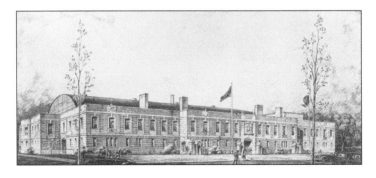

Architect's rendering of the new Fort York Armoury (77).

(from left to right): the Irish Regiment ("*Fiord Go Bas,*" Gaelic for "Faithful Unto Death"), the Queen's York Rangers, the Royal Regiment of Canada ("*Nec Aspera Terrant,*" Latin for "We Fear No Hardships") and the Toronto Scottish Regiment. The building's cornerstone, dated 1933, can be found at the southwest corner. The facility remains in active use with four of the original five units still calling the place home. The Irish Regiment moved out and was replaced by the 709th (Reserve) Communications Regiment.

CORONATION PARK (78): On the same day that King George VI was crowned in England, May 12, 1937, the City of Toronto officially dedicated a newly created waterfront park to be known as Coronation Park. As part of the dedication ceremony, 149 maple trees and one royal oak were planted in the park to commemorate the 150 units of the Canadian Expeditionary Force that participated in the First World War. Two years later, during the visit to our city by the King and his Queen, 123 more trees were planted, one for each public and separate school in Toronto. In 1958, Coronation Park became part of Exhibition Park and eight years later, along with the entire CNE grounds, became the responsibility of the Metropolitan (now) Toronto Parks Department. In 1995, a new memorial in the form of a 120-foot flagpole and sculpture by John McEwen that together commemorate the fiftieth anniversary of the end of the Second World War was unveiled in the park. The wording surrounding the sculpture represents the word "Peace" in fifty different languages.

SECOND INVASION OF YORK (site of, 79): War between Britain and the United States broke out on June 18, 1812, with towns on either side of Lakes Ontario and Erie becoming battlegrounds on several occasions. One of these conflicts, which in reality was a very one-sided skirmish, occurred on July 31, 1813, more than a century before landfilling removed Fort York from the water's edge. On that date a number of American troops carried out a second attack on York (Toronto). Unlike the first American occupation earlier in the year, which lasted a total of five days (see 117) there were no British troops in town to help repel the invaders. However, this time the small American detachment departed the town after just three days, having burned the storehouse at Gibraltar Point on the Peninsula (now Toronto Island) and the barracks at Fort York. The historic plaque erected in Coronation Park marks the approximate location of where the American ships entered Toronto Bay those many years ago.

*   *   *   *   *

AVRO LANCASTER BOMBER (80): Work on the Canadian-built version of the famous British Lancaster bomber began at the Victory Aircraft Ltd. factory at Malton, northwest of Toronto, in early 1943 with the first prototype, KB700, flown over Toronto on August 1, 1943. A total of 229 Lancasters were built at the Malton plant during the period July, 1943, to September, 1945. This "Lanc" was built in 1945 and designated FM-104. It operated as a search and rescue aircraft out of Torbay, Newfoundland, until it was retired in 1964 and put on display. As this book was being written a more secure site for this Toronto "artifact" was being sought.

## Cross Lake Shore Boulevard, proceed east on Fleet Street then under the archway and north on Garrison Road

FORT YORK (81): One of the first things Lieutenant-Governor John Graves Simcoe did in the process of establishing his new capital at York (Toronto) was to build a fort to defend the small townsite, several miles to the east, from attack. In those far-off days the Peninsula (now Toronto Island) was connected to the mainland at its easternmost end by a narrow isthmus (see Ward's Island). As a result the only entrance into the harbour was through the old Western Gap. To protect this entrance Simcoe decided to build a fort on the water's edge with its cannons ready to batter any enemy craft attempting to enter the bay. As a result of numerous landfilling projects the fort appears today to have been built well inland. Fort York, which dates from 1793, was attacked by American forces twice during the War of 1812 and many of the structures were destroyed. Well-known American general and explorer Zebulon Montgomery Pike, who in 1806 discovered what is now called Pike's Peak in the Front Range of the Rocky Mountains in Colorado, was killed during an attack on Fort York on April 27, 1813. Following the war, much of the fort was rebuilt, but soon fell into disuse when a "new" fort, now Stanley Barracks, was built in 1841 (see 88). Then, as part of the city's centennial celebrations in 1934, "old" Fort York was restored and today, as an extremely active Heritage Toronto site, it is one of the city's most popular attractions. It is located on Garrison Road north of the former Molson brewery building.

\*   \*   \*   \*   \*

## Return to Fleet Street and proceed west

STRACHAN AVENUE: Named for the Honourable and Reverend John Strachan (1778–1867), one of the most influential people in the early days of our city. Strachan was born in Aberdeen, Scotland and came to Upper Canada (Ontario) in 1799 where he obtained a teaching position in Kingston at an annual salary of $400. He was ordained an Anglican priest in 1804 and eight years later moved with his family to York (Toronto) where he was appointed Rector of St. James' Church, the town's first church established just five years earlier. During the occupation of the little town by American forces in 1813, Strachan was front and centre in ensuring proper treatment of the citizens by the invaders. In 1839, Strachan became Bishop of Toronto and in 1850 was instrumental in the establishment of Trinity College, a university controlled by his Anglican Church. The first Trinity College was erected on Queen Street West and the street leading to it was named Strachan Avenue in memory of its founder who died in his 90th year and was given a state funeral by the citizens of a greatful city. Trinity is now affiliated with the University of Toronto and is located on Hoskin Avenue near Queen's Park. Strachan's original Trinity College was demolished in 1956. Only the college's impressive gates remain.

## Proceed north on Strachan Avenue

MILITARY BURIAL GROUNDS (82): Located on the east side of Strachan Avenue just north of Fleet Street and on part of the historic Garrison Reserve set aside by Governor Simcoe for military purposes is the small Military Burial Grounds or, more correctly, the Garrison Cemetery, where the first interments occurred in the 1830s. This cemetery was the final resting place for hundreds of officers and men (and their families) of a dozen British line regiments and Canadian units stationed in Toronto. A few decipherable headstones remain though hundreds of soldiers rest in unmarked graves. The last dated interment was in 1927.

\*　\*　\*　\*　\*

# Return to Lake Shore Boulevard, enter the Exhibition Grounds through the Princes' Gate and proceed west on Princes' Boulevard

## Exhibition Place (83) (* indicates Exhibition Place sites):

The area that today is referred to as Exhibition Place grew out of an arrangement drawn up between the city and federal governments in 1878 whereby Toronto became

> the lessee for a term of twenty years, renewable, at a rental of $100 per year, of all of the westerly portion of the Garrison Common containing 51 3/4 acres and also a roadway 66 feet wide leading thereto from Strachan Avenue. This land is to be used as an Exhibition Park and as a place for the Provincial, County and several Electoral Division and Township Exhibitions of Agricultural products, Arts and Manufacturers, under the management of the several Associations organized by Act of Parliament and also for Horticultural and other exhibitions or purposes as may, from time to time be authorized, ordered or permitted by resolution of the City Council.

Later that same year, the 1878 edition of the Provincial Exhibition was held in this newly acquired Exhibition Park. An attempt was then made by the city to have all succeeding Provincial Exhibitions held in Toronto, but the governing body said no. So, early in 1879, a new society called the Industrial Exhibition Association of Toronto was formed and in September of 1879, held its first fair, a three-week-long event in Exhibition Park that featured 8,234 exhibits and welcomed over 100,000 visitors each of whom paid a twenty-five-cent admission fee. Since that first successful year, the Canadian National Exhibition (so called, officially, since 1904) has been held annually except for the period 1942 to 1946 when the park and buildings were taken over by the government for military purposes. The Ex, as it's affectionately known, has grown into one of the largest annual exhibitions in the world. Exhibition Park, now called Exhibition Place, is also home to the Royal Agricultural Winter Fair, the Sportsmen's Show, and numerous other trade and public events. Until SkyDome opened in 1989 the CNE Grandstand was home to both the Blue Jay baseball and Argonaut football teams. Some of the most interesting features of the grounds are the numerous old buildings and other structures that have been erected over the years.

\* PRINCES' GATES, 1927 (84): Originally called the Diamond Jubilee of Confederation Gates, to commemorate the sixtieth anniversary of Canada's birth, and built in just 4 1/2 months at a cost of $152,240.47, this impressive structure, stretching 350 feet (107 metres) from end to end, was renamed the Princes' Gates soon after its dedication by Edward, the Prince of Wales, and his brother Prince George on August 30, 1927. The centre arch is topped by a 24-foot (7-metre) concrete statue of Winged Victory, who represents progress and advance. The present statue was cast out of an advanced plastic composite material in mid-1987 to replace the severely damaged original. The statue is surrounded by sculptured embellishments created by Charles McKechnie that represent music, education, and the arts. The architect of the Gates was Alfred Chapman, who is also responsible for the Ontario Government Building (see 108) at the west end of the grounds.

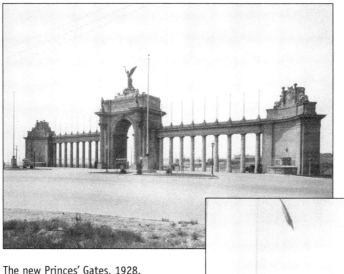

The new Princes' Gates, 1928.

The elder prince cuts the ribbon during the dedication proceedings, August 30, 1927.

* AUTOMOTIVE BUILDING, 1929 (85): This magnificent structure, designed by Canadian architect Douglas Kertland, was where Exhibition visitors got to see the newest cars and trucks each fall. As vehicle model introduction dates changed, the structure began filling a new role as a major exhibition building, a role it continues to this day. During the Second World War, the building was used by members of the Royal Canadian Navy and known affectionately (or not) as the HMCS Auto Building. The Automotive Building is now connected with the Trade Centre across Princes' Boulevard by an underground tunnel.

* NATIONAL TRADE CENTRE, 1997 (86): One of the reasons for the creation of the Toronto Industrial Exhibition (and its successor, the Canadian National Exhibition) was to promote the idea of trade. In fact, it wasn't far from the site of this new trade centre that the native Canadians traded with the French nearly two-and-a-half centuries ago (see 101). Ground breaking for the $180 million National Trade Centre took place on June 28, 1995 with construction completed early in 1997. The official opening was held on April 3 and the first event in the new building was the 1997 edition of the National Home Show. The massive building with all manner of state-of-the-art features contains in excess of 700,000 square feet of covered space that, when combined with the adjacent Coliseum (to which it is connected by a glass-covered atrium and the Automotive Building, accessed via an underground walkway), gives a total of more than one million square feet of rentable space. The building also features underground parking for almost 1,300 cars. An interesting feature of the new building is the way in which the Princes' Boulevard facade has been treated architecturally. The east end appears to mirror the classic appearance of the 1929 Automotive Building on the south side of the street. As one proceeds further west, the centre changes face, taking on a much more futuristic look.

* COLISEUM (87): Tucked in behind and attached to the Trade Centre by Heritage Court is the Coliseum. Designed by G.W.F. Price of the City Architect's Department, the $1.3-million structure was built in conjunction with the Royal Winter Fair, which held its inaugural event in the new building in 1922. When it opened, the Coliseum had the largest floor space under one roof anywhere in the world. Interestingly, the building was originally designed with the main entrance facing north to take advantage of the proposed new streetcar line that was to be laid down along the street behind it. That line didn't materialize until 1996. The Livestock Pavilion Annex to the east was erected at a cost of $750,000 in 1926. The Coliseum complex was "home" to thousands of airmen during the Second World War. When the Trade Centre was first proposed it was decided to use

a covered court to connect it with the Coliseum. A number of sculptures saved from old, now-demolished Exhibition buildings have been preserved in Heritage Court.

   * Former STANLEY BARRACKS (88): Erected in 1841 by the Royal Engineers as the Officers' Quarters, this structure is the only building still standing of the many that made up the "new" fort (as opposed to the "old" Fort York). The name was eventually changed to commemorate Frederick Arthur Stanley, Lord Stanley, the country's sixth governor general who served from 1888 to 1893. This is the same gentleman who, in 1894, donated the Stanley Cup which is now awarded to the top team in the National Hockey League. In more recent years, this historic building has been the home of the Canadian Sports Hall of Fame, Melody Fair, and until recently, the Marine Museum of Upper Canada. Just to the east of the Marine Museum is the Montreal-built 627,000 lb. (284,400 kg) "Northern" class steam locomotive #6213 built for Canadian National Railways in 1942. Old #6213 operated on various routes across Canada until retired and donated to the citizens of Toronto in 1960.

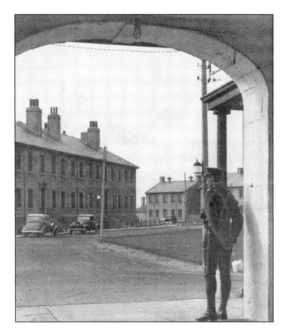

The building on the left is the sole survivor of the Stanley Barracks complex, 1932.

# Cross bridge to Ontario Place

## Ontario Place (89):

This internationally acclaimed cultural, leisure time, and entertainment complex was initiated by the late John Robarts, the premier of Ontario from 1961 to 1971. The project actually materialized as a result of Toronto's bid to host the 1976 Summer Olympic Games, a bid that died when the event was awarded to Montreal. The money that was to be invested in turning the Exhibition grounds into an Olympic site, some $15 million, went to build Ontario Place instead. Ontario Place covers 96 acres (38 hectares) of man-made islands, the creation of which required more than 2.5 million cubic yards (1.53 cubic metres) of clean fill, much of which came from the construction of the TTC's Bloor-Danforth subway. To protect these islands from the frequently turbulent waters of Lake Ontario, three large retired lake freighters, *Douglas Houghton, Victorious,* and *Howard L. Shaw* were filled with concrete and sunk along the south promenade of Ontario Place forming a seawall 1,320 feet (402 metres) in length. The $29-million Ontario Place complex was officially opened on May 22, 1971.

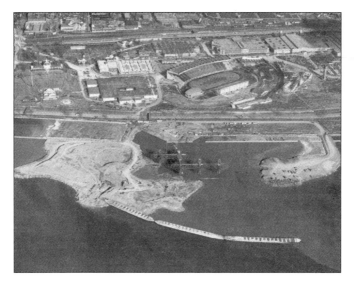

Ontario Place begins to take shape., 1970. The three former lake freighters that form the breakwall are also visible.

HMCS *HAIDA*, one of Ontario Place's feature attractions, has a history of its own. This 375-foot (114-metre) "Tribal" class destroyer was built in Britain for the Royal Canadian Navy and commissioned on August 30, 1943. *Haida*, and her crew of 250, spent much of their time on convoy duty between various English ports and Murmansk in Russia. Later *Haida* patrolled the English Channel where she sank several enemy ships and rescued some of the crew of her stricken sister ship, HMCS *Athabaskan*, sunk by a torpedo from a German destroyer on April 28, 1944. *Haida* also had a tour of duty with the NATO forces during the Korean conflict (1950–1953). Canada's "fightingest" ship was decommissioned in October of 1963. It was saved from the scrapyard when it was purchased by a group of interested citizens. *Haida* has been a feature of Ontario Place since the attraction's opening in 1971. Other attractions include the Cinesphere Imax Theatre, Children's Village, Lego Creative Play Centre, the nine-thousand-seat (sixteen thousand with grass seating) Molson Amphitheatre, Sea Trek simulator ride, Atlantis entertainment and restaurant complex, the Island Club/Island Stage, Thrill Zone Game Pod plus many others — too many to list. In addition there are rides for all ages, fast food and family restaurants, and gift and specialty shops. Call (416)314-9900 for recorded information. Ontario Place is open to the public from mid-May until mid-September.

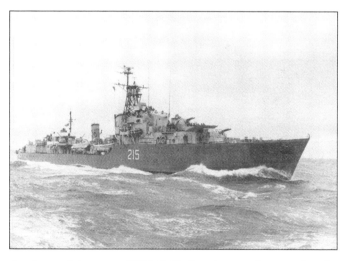

A veteran of two wars, HMCS *Haida* found a new home at Ontario Place in 1971.

## Return to the Exhibition Grounds
## and proceed west on Princes' Boulevard

## Exhibition Place [continued]:

* HORSE PALACE, 1931 (90): City Architect J.J. Woolnough was responsible for this $1-million structure with the money coming from all three levels of government: federal, provincial, and municipal. This unique structure is used during the Ex, the Royal Winter Fair, and other public events that feature horse shows. During the Second World War, the Palace was a manning depot for the Canadian army.

* EXHIBITION STADIUM (91): This stadium was the fourth such facility to be erected on this site. The covered portion was erected in 1947 with the south stands added in the mid-1970s. From 1959 until 1989, the 54,500-seat stadium was home to the Canadian Football League Toronto Argonauts (see 111) and, in 1977, the Toronto Blue Jays of the American League, made their debut at Exhibition Stadium with a 9–5 win over the Chicago White Sox before a crowd of 44,649. On several occasions during the summer months, as well as on most evenings of the annual Canadian National Exhibition, a portable stage was rolled into place in front of the north stands and "big name" grandstand shows were presented. The largest crowd to ever attend an event at Exhibition Stadium occurred in 1980 when seventy thousand fans attended "The Who" concert. Plans announced in early 1998 called for the grandstand to be demolished at the conclusion of that year's annual Exhibition.

* CANADA'S SPORTS HALL OF FAME (92): Originally this building housed the Hockey Hall of Fame when it opened in 1961. The building was enlarged and in 1967 the Canadian Sports Hall of Fame moved into the east end of the building. The Hockey Hall of Fame is now located in the former Bank of Montreal building at the northwest corner of Yonge and Front streets.

* FOOD BUILDING (93): The most popular building during the annual Exhibition is this structure, which opened in 1954.

* QUEEN ELIZABETH EXHIBIT HALL AND THEATRE (94): Completed in 1957 and used for various events year round. The Administration Offices for both Exhibition Place and the annual Canadian National Exhibition are located at the west end of this complex.

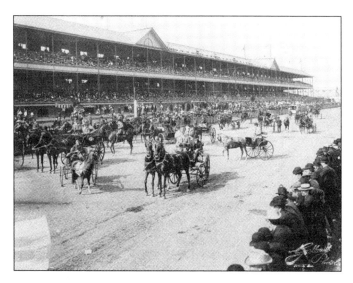

The original Exhibition grandstand circa 1900.

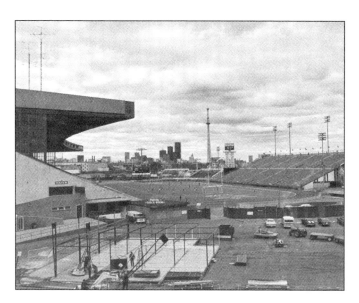

CNE Stadium in the mid-1970s. Note the still unfinished CN Tower (47), and the now demolished Shell Tower, in the centre distance.

* BETTER LIVING CENTRE (95): Built in 1962 on the site of the 1903 Manufacturers Building, which was destroyed by fire in 1961, this unheated, non-air-conditioned building's primary use is during the twenty-day CNE, though it is used on occasion for other events during the warmer months.

* Former RAILWAYS BUILDINGS, later MUSIC BUILDING (96): Erected in 1908, this unique structure, with its three exhibit halls for the three national railways of the day, has featured many kinds of attractions over the years. Best remembered are Hydroscope (where the plans for the St. Lawrence Seaway were introduced to the public) and Vetascope (where visitors could watch a calf being born in the so-called Moo-ternity Ward). For many years the building became the Music Building and various musical programmes were featured in what were converted into small concert halls. In recent years the building, which suffered serious damage as a result of a fire, has been used for a variety of purposes.

* The CNE FIREHALL (97) was designed by architect George Gouinlock and was first placed in service for the 1912 Exhibition. Originally housing horse-drawn equipment, the Exhibition Hall is only used during the twenty days of the annual fair.

* Former ADMINISTRATION BUILDING, now PRESS BUILDING (98): For many years after it opened in 1905, this handsome structure, designed by the CNE's architect George Gouinlock and built at a cost of $15,000 (!), housed the annual Exhibition's Administrative Offices with the Canadian National Exhibition Association's board and dining rooms on the second floor. The building now houses Exhibition offices.

* HORTICULTURAL BUILDING (99): Erected in 1907 on the site of the Exhibition's first permanent building, the Crystal Palace, which was destroyed by fire a year earlier, this beautiful building was designed by CNE architect George Gouinlock. It is basically a "twenty-day" building, but in September of 1949 the Horticultural Building was pressed into use as a temporary morgue for the identification of victims of the *Noronic* disaster (see 25).

* BANDSHELL (100): Erected in time for the 1936 CNE, this unique structure continues in use every Exhibition and people still marvel at its marvellous acoustical properties.

* Site of FORT ROUILLÉ (101): The large obelisk flanked by two cannons just to the west of the bandshell commemorates the approximate site of a French fort established in 1750 to intercept the Mississauga Indians, who descended the nearby Humber River with their furs and

crossed Lake Ontario to trade with the enemy of the French, the English who had several trading posts throughout what is now New York State. The fort was commissioned by Antoine Louis Rouillé, the French colonial minister, for whom the fort was officially named though it was more frequently called Fort Toronto after the surrounding area. For nine years, the fort's commandant and his men where kept busy, but three years after the Seven Years' War between England and France broke out in 1756, the little fort was burned to prevent it from falling into the hands of the English. The site was excavated in 1984 as part of the city's 150th anniversary celebrations. The wooden walls of the fort were outlined in stone and an explanatory plaque erected.

* LAKE SHORE BOULEVARD BAILEY BRIDGE (102): Erected in 1947 to permit pedestrian access to the waterfront, this Bailey bridge is but one of thousands of similar structures all over the world that were built to the design of engineering wizard Donald Coleman Bailey. Bailey, who was an engineer in the British Ministry of Supply during the Second World War, designed an open lattice-work bridge that was both light and portable yet strong enough to permit heavy tanks and trucks to cross. Hundreds were erected throughout the various theatres of war. For his efforts, Mr. Donald Bailey became Sir Donald Bailey in 1945. How did this one arrive here in Toronto? Prior to the outbreak of the Second World War, traffic on Lake Shore Boulevard was light enough to simply detour cars and trucks around the grounds during the period of the fair. Following the war, the increased traffic on the Lake Shore made crossing the thoroughfare on foot extremely dangerous. This type of bridge was found to be perfect to get visitors to the first post-war edition of the Canadian National Exhibition, held in 1947, to and from the activities on the waterfront in safety.

* SCADDING CABIN (103): Built in 1796 by John Scadding, one of our community's earliest settlers, the little Scadding Cabin originally stood on the east bank of the Don River north of Queen Street. It was moved by a group of York Pioneers to its present location at Exhibition Place in the Ex's first year, 1879. The York Pioneers and Historical Society continue to look after this historic structure.

* CNE FLAGPOLE (104): Just north of the Fort Rouillé monument is the CNE's main flagpole. This magnificent 185-foot (56-metre) pole was shaped from a Vancouver Island, British Columbia Douglas fir that had been toppled in a fierce wind storm. With financial assistance from Travel South, an organization of tourist associations representing states in the southeastern part of the U.S.A., the new pole was erected on this site in time for the 1977 edition of the Exhibition.

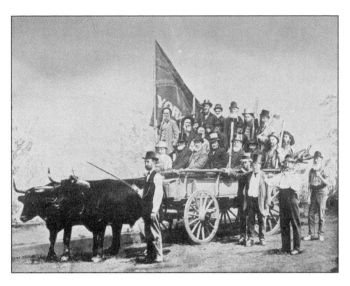

A group of York Pioneers on their way to the Exhibition to reconstruct the Scadding Cabin (103).

* Former DOMINION GOVERNMENT BUILDING, later ARTS, CRAFTS AND HOBBIES BUILDING, now the location of MEDIEVAL TIMES DINNER AND TOURNAMENT (105): This striking building was erected in 1912 to a design of the CNE's architect George Gouinlock, who is also responsible for the nearby Horticultural, Press, and Railway buildings. Built at a cost of $125,000 the structure was originally used as a display hall by a multitude of foreign governments as well as by provincial authorities during the run of the annual CNE. In later years it was devoted to other displays such as those of artisans, crafts people and hobbyists. In the summer of 1993, major interior changes were made and an addition constructed at the west end of the structure. Today the historic building is home to a year-round attraction called Medieval Times Dinner and Tournament.

* CENTENNIAL SQUARE (106), which includes the small bandshell, a reproduction of the one that stood south of the Horticultural Building, was built to commemorate the CNE's centennial year. The first phase, the bandstand and the north-south leg opened in 1978, the year the one hundredth edition of the annual fair took place. The east-west leg opened one year later. In recent years the square has been whittled down so that now only the bandstand and east-west leg remain.

* DUFFERIN GATE (107): This structure was erected in 1960 and replaced an older, more impressive looking gate that was demolished when the Gardiner Expressway was built north of the Exhibition Grounds.

* DUFFERIN STREET: Named for Frederick Temple Hamilton-Temple-Blackwood, Lord Dufferin, Governor General of Canada who served from 1872–1878. In retrospect, it's fitting that the main thoroughfare into the west end of the Canadian National Exhibition grounds is named in honour of the Queen's representative in Canada, a man who was in office at the very time the Exhibition was being promoted by local politicians and influential businessmen.

* Former ONTARIO GOVERNMENT BUILDING (108): This unique structure, built at a cost of $600,000, was a contribution of the provincial government to the CNE in 1926. For many years, the province featured marvellous exhibits in this building that depicted all regions of Ontario. However, when the province built Ontario Place across the Lake Shore in the early 1970s, they simply abandoned the building. It eventually became the Carlsberg Building and in recent years the home of the CNE Casino.

## Proceed west on British Columbia Drive then cross to south side of Lake Shore Boulevard

MARILYN BELL PARK (109): This park was named during Toronto's 150th birthday celebrations in 1984 for the first person to successfully swim across Lake Ontario. Marilyn was born in Toronto in 1937 and after living for a time in North Bay, Ontario, and Halifax, Nova Scotia, Marilyn returned to Toronto with her family following the end of the Second World War. She joined Gus Ryder's swimming club and trained, first in the Oakwood Swimming Pool and later in the Credit River east of Toronto. As a young girl, Marilyn won her first major swimming competitions in the lake south of the Canadian National Exhibition Grounds. In September of 1954, she was selected as a substitute member of a team of four men competing in that year's Canadian National Exhibition cross-lake marathon swim. Rather than being just a substitute swimmer, the 16-year-old schoolgirl decided to attempt the entire 32-mile (51.5-kilometre) crossing from Youngstown in New York State to the Exhibition waterfront. If successful, she would become the first person in history to succeed in this gruelling feat. Entering the water at 11:07 p.m. on September 8, 1954, and battling eels, cold water, nausea, and tremendous odds for the next twenty hours and fifty-seven minutes, an exhausted Marilyn touched the breakwall in front of the Boulevard Club (see 114) to the cheers of tens of thousands

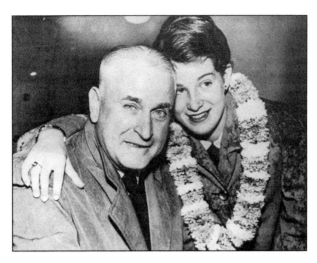

The first "lady of the lake," Marilyn Bell (109) with her coach Gus Ryder (124).

of Torontonians gathered along he city's waterfront. A collective sigh of relief swept across the country. Our Marilyn had done it! In 1955, Marilyn successfully swam the English Channel and in 1956, the treacherous Straits of Juan de Fuca located between Vancouver Island and the United States mainland. Today, Marilyn Bell DiLascio, mother, grandmother, and wife, lives with her husband Joseph in New Jersey.

WESTERN BREAKWALL (110): As part of the overall waterfront redevelopment plan proposed by the Toronto Harbour Commission in 1912, it was felt imperative that a breakwater be constructed to protect the city's western beaches from erosion and to provide a protected waterway for small craft. The Western Breakwall project, which was to be paid for by the federal government, was approved in 1913 and work was underway when the Great War broke out. Dozens of wooden cribs fabricated out of 12-inch-square (4.7-metre-square) timbers were sunk to bedrock 350 feet (107 metres) south of the newly created shoreline and filled with ballast stone. Next, precast concrete blocks were placed on top of the cribs until the blocks protruded above the waterline. A deck of poured concrete was then applied with a sloping face to deflect the incoming waves. Following the end of the war, work resumed on the Western Breakwall (also known as the Government Breakwater since they paid for it), and by the end of 1924 all 17,985 feet (5,482 metres) of breakwall, from the Humber River to the Western Gap, were in place.

JAMESON AVENUE: Born in Harbridge, England, Robert Sympson Jameson (1796–1854) was called to the bar in 1823 and six years later became the Chief Justice of Dominica in the West Indies. Unhappy in that position, he was soon made attorney general of Upper Canada (Ontario) in 1833 (the last provincial attorney general to be appointed to the position by the British government) and four years later became the Vice-Chancellor of the Court of Chancery, an important judicial position that he fulfilled with great skill. Jameson also served on numerous government boards and was extremely active socially, being a founder of the St. George's Society, the Toronto Literary Club, the Toronto Society of Arts, and the Church of St. George the Martyr. Jameson married, and was subsequently separated from, Anna (Murphy) Jameson, whose 1838 book *Winter Studies and Summer Rambles in Canada* gives a fascinating view of our country as it was a century-and-a-half ago. Though Jameson's life appears to have been one of great fulfilment, he died in Toronto an unhappy man. The present Jameson Avenue was so named since this prominent Torontonian owned property in the area.

ARGONAUT ROWING CLUB, 1225 Lake Shore Boulevard West (111): Established in 1872 in a small clubhouse overlooking Toronto Bay at the foot of George Street, the Argonaut Rowing Club is the longest continuously operating rowing club in the country. The club eventually moved a little further west to the end of a pier at the foot of York Street alongside a number of other aquatic clubs. As the waterfront redevelopment got closer to the York Street pier, it was time to move again. A new building was then erected at the foot of Jameson Avenue (when that street used to run right down to the water's edge) and after that structure burned in early 1947, the present clubhouse was built as a replacement on the same site. In the early years of the Argonaut Rowing Club, an amateur football team was organized. Eventually, this team evolved into a major league professional team known as the Toronto Argonauts. Interestingly, when the rights to the name "Argonauts" were purchased from the rowing club in the early 1950s, part of the money realized from the sale was used to construct a second floor on the present clubhouse.

DOWLING AVENUE: Colonel Dowling was the brother-in-law of Alexander Roberts Dunn, the first Canadian-born recipient of the Victoria Cross. The young Dunn won the coveted medal during the Crimean War's Battle of Balaclava, October 25, 1854. Colonel Dowling had married Dunn's sister thereby becoming the son-in-law of John Henry Dunn, the receiver-general of Canada from 1820 to 1844, who owned property in the area. It was only fitting, therefore, that the two nearby streets, Dowling and Dunn, be named for members of the Dunn family.

TORONTO SAILING AND CANOE CLUB, 1391 Lake Shore Boulevard West (112): This extremely active waterfront club was established in 1880 by a group of nine prominent Toronto businessmen. Five years passed before the young club was able to move into their first rented clubhouse located on the bayfront west of the foot of Bay Street. Two years later, in 1887, the membership had grown so quickly that a new facility was necessary. A new clubhouse was erected on the shoreline a little further west and just south of the Union Station of the day (the station would have been at the foot of today's University Avenue) and sufficed for the next six years until another move saw the popular canoe club in a new and larger building on a pier at the foot of York Street. By 1909, the club's membership had grown to almost six hundred. Then, as happened with other bayfront residents when the Harbour Commission began redeveloping the central waterfront in the early 1920s, another new site for the clubhouse became necessary. The club purchased the former McGann Estate just west of the foot of today's Dowling Avenue (at that time all the north-south streets in the area ran down to the water's edge) and moved into an old house on the property. By the end of the 1920s, the club had run into serious financial difficulties and was forced to sell most of their property. They were able to retain the old boathouse and this became their clubhouse. In 1939, the Toronto Canoe Club was renamed the Toronto Sailing and Canoe Club. The membership was dealt a severe blow on February 22, 1957, when fire destroyed much of the old clubhouse including almost one hundred dinghies and canoes stored in the structure. After months of negotiations, during which time the unburned part of the clubhouse was used for meetings, city council loaned the club sufficient money to help construct the present building, which opened in 1960. Today, club membership numbers close to 350 people who sail a variety of craft measuring from 13 to 33 feet (4 to 10 metres) in length. Interestingly though, there are no more canoes at the Toronto Canoe Club.

ROYAL CANADIAN LEGION QUEEN'S OWN RIFLES BRANCH 344, 1395 Lake Shore Boulevard West (113): This building was built in 1927 as the headquarters of the Navy League of Canada. A portion of the inscription on the commemorative plaque unveiled at the official opening by the then-premier of the province of Ontario, Howard Ferguson (and visible at the northeast corner of the building), reads "This building was erected in the interest of all British seamen upon whom, in no mean measure, depend the safety, the preservation and the prosperity of the Empire." In its early years, this building was also the headquarters of the Sea Cadets Corps and the Toronto Half-Company of the Royal Canadian Navy Volunteer Reserve which eventually became HMCS York (see 76). In more recent years, the building has been home to the Rameses Shrine and, since

1983, to the 550 or so members of the Royal Canadian Legion's Branch 344. The Legion, of which there are more than 1,800 branches in Canada and the United States, is an organization for ex-servicemen and women and was established in 1925 in Winnipeg, Manitoba.

BOULEVARD CLUB, 1491 Lake Shore Boulevard West (114): Established in 1905 as the Parkdale Canoe Club (the initials PCC are still visible on the north side of the present building), the club's first meetings were held in a parlour at the rear of Mrs. Meyer's Restaurant, which was located on the waterfront just west of the present Boulevard Club site. Soon the forty-three club members had raised enough money to build their first clubhouse. Unfortunately, the little wooden building burned soon after it opened. Then, before a replacement structure could be completed, it too burned. Another new clubhouse, erected at the end of a long pier jutting into the lake, was ready in time for the 1915 season. Eight years later, with a club membership of 1,200, fire struck again. The following year, 1924, saw a fourth clubhouse erected on the same site only now, with acres of land having been reclaimed for the new Sunnyside bathing beaches, this building sat high and dry. It is this clubhouse, though much expanded, that remains in use today. The name Parkdale Canoe Club (Parkdale was the nearby town, and the neighbourhood north of the clubhouse retains the name) was changed to Boulevard Club in 1935. A swimming pool was added in the mid-1930s, curling introduced in 1957, and seven years later a separate boathouse was built. Major renovations were undertaken in 1968 and two years later the huge bubble in front of the main building, which now covers seven tennis courts, was added. Today, several thousand members enjoy sailing, curling, tennis, lawn bowling, and numerous other activities at the Boulevard Club.

The collection of HILLSIDE LOGOS (115), a unique feature of the city stretching along the embankment north of Lake Shore Boulevard, the Gardiner Expressway, and the railway corridor, was the creation of a local company, Hillside Communications, with the first of the logos appearing in 1987. Their placement required the approval of two civic departments as well as the blessing of Canadian National, owners of the corridor, followed by the removal of more than twelve tons of garbage from a busy part of the corridor that had become a real eyesore. Today there are fourteen logos, eleven representing corporations, two devoted to charities (presently the United Way and the Toronto Symphony Orchestra) and one, the centrepiece, set aside for the City of Toronto. Each spring 20,000 daffodils bring a splash of colour to the once-drab hillside while 23,000 coloured lights illuminate the setting every Christmas. The number of plants used in the landscaping of the logos is in excess of 65,000.

GO TRANSIT (116): Frequently seen operating over the aforementioned rail corridor are the trains of GO Transit, an interregional transit operation set up by the Government of Ontario (thus the title "GO"), that provides commuter service to and from the numerous communities within a 50-mile (80-kilometre) radius of Toronto. GO Transit rail service, with a single rail line, was established as a three-year experimental project on May 23, 1967. The concept flourished with today's operations well in excess of all predictions. In 1970 a commuter bus service was added. The unique green and white bi-level rail passenger coaches, built at the Hawker Siddeley plant in Thunder Bay, Ontario, were introduced in 1978. Presently, service is offered over seven rail corridors with a total of 139 weekday train trips over 361 kilometres serving 49 stations. In addition there are six bus corridors with 1,000 weekday bus trips over 1,235 kilometres to 13 terminals. GO's equipment fleet consists of 49 locomotives and 131 bi-level rail coaches plus 184 buses. Approximately 120,000 passengers (91,000 on trains, 29,000 on buses) use the various GO Transit routes daily. In the first year of operations GO Transit carried 2.5 million passengers. Today the combined bus and rail system carries almost 34 million riders annually. Incidentally, the rail corridor follows a route pioneered by the Great Western Railway back in 1855 and realigned in a grade-separated cut (a right-of-way cut into the embankment) earlier this century. Today, in addition to the GO trains, a variety of freight services operate over this track as well as intercity and transcontinental passenger trains operated by VIA Rail Canada Ltd. VIA was established as a Crown Corporation in 1978, after a brief time as a subsidiary of CN, and operates all passenger train service in the country.

AMERICAN INVASION OF YORK, 1813 (site of, 117): War between the United States and Great Britain broke out June 18, 1812. Several major battles ensued including those at Detroit and Queenston Heights, with the British claiming victories in both. Eventually an attempt was made by American forces to capture the provincial capital at York and it was in this general vicinity that on April 27, 1813, some 1,700 American troops stormed ashore and, after battling British regulars and a few local militia and Indians, attacked Fort York (see 81) several miles to the east. The Town of York quickly fell and for almost a week what is now the City of Toronto was an American possession. York was again attacked, though less forcefully, later that same year (see 79). In the summer of 1814, British troops overran Washington, D.C. and on August 24, 1814, did the unthinkable. As described in a British general's diary, the "red coats" set fire to the so-called President's Mansion "in direct retaliation for the destruction of York's public buildings" the previous year. After the invaders had retired whitewash was applied to the building to cover the unsightly expanse of charred wood, and before long the locals began referring to the residence the "White House." Teddy Roosevelt made it official during his term of office by placing those words at the top of the presidential stationery.

PALAIS ROYALE, 1601 Lake Shore Boulevard West (118): One of only three landmarks that remains from the magical days of Sunnyside Amusement Park, the Palais Royale dance hall was erected in 1920 at a cost of $60,000. At first it was simply Dean's Boathouse where the famous Sunnyside Torpedo Canoe and Sunnyside Cruiser were built and sold, complete with lessons on how to get the most out of your purchase. This marketing strategy didn't work that well, for soon Mr. Dean was in financial trouble. Within a few months the Palais Royale dance hall opened in the building and this new addition to the popular Sunnyside amusement park on the waterfront was an immediate success. In no time the biggest of the big bands were "swinging and swaying," "knocking 'em dead," and fans were "jumpin' and jivin'" at the Palais Royale. Two of Toronto's own home-grown bands were popular attractions at the Palais in their own right. The bands of Bert Niosi and Ellis McLintock were as good as any that played at Sunnyside. Now, many years later, the Palais Royale lives on with the big bands of today appearing almost every weekend.

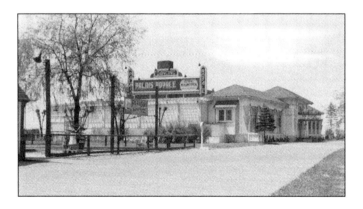

The still-popular Palais Royale dance hall when it was on the boardwalk at Sunnyside Amusement Park, circa 1950.

\* \* \* \* \*

PEDESTRIAN FOOTBRIDGE (119): Before the construction of the Gardiner Expressway in the late 1950s, pedestrian access to the waterfront was easy. In fact, until the construction of Lake Shore Boulevard in the 1920s, many of the tree-lined side streets in the neighbourhood ran from King Street right to the water's edge. But with the arrival of the limited-access Gardiner Expressway in the mid-1950s, the Parkdale community was totally cut off from its beach. So, in 1958, the city constructed this $250,000 footbridge high above twelve lanes of traffic and four pairs of railway tracks. Now, it's the only pedestrian link to the waterfront between Parkside Avenue to the west and Dowling Avenue to the east.

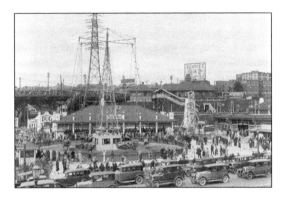

Some of the rides at Sunnyside, the train station and busy King, Queen, Roncesvalles, and Lakeshore Road intersection on the hill in the background, 1929.

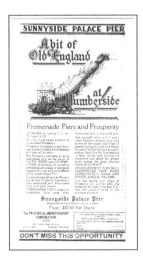

Promotional ad for Toronto's new Palace Pier at the mouth of the Humber River, 1928.

SUNNYSIDE AMUSEMENT PARK (site of, 120): As part of the massive waterfront redevelopment plan of 1912, the Toronto Harbour Commission decided to build an amusement park on the site of the old Humber Bay at the western approach to the city. New land for the park was created using fill pumped from the lake bottom just offshore by huge dredges. On June 28, 1922, Sunnyside Amusement park was officially opened by the mayor of the day, Alfred McGuire. The 15 1/2 acres (6 hectares) of rides, restaurants, games, and dance halls soon became known as "the poor man's Riviera" and thousands of men, women, and children flocked to the park almost every day and night for the next thirty-three years. Sing-alongs, boat burnings, dance marathons, parachute jumping exhibitions, old car contests, and people like Shipwreck Kelly, world champion flagpole sitter, proved to be popular attractions as well. When one speaks of attractions, one of the greatest crowd pleasers was the Miss Toronto Contest sponsored, in those days, by the people who ran Sunnyside. The first Miss Toronto contest was held at Sunnyside in 1926 with pretty Jean Tolmie selected as the winner. Another event held annually for many years at Sunnyside was the extremely popular Easter Parade during which hundreds of people, dressed in their finest attire, would parade along the park's 24-foot-wide (7.3 metres), mile-and-a-half-long (2,440 metres) wooden boardwalk (usually defying a cold wind off the lake) which was constructed by the Harbour Commission between the traffic boulevard and the new bathing beach. For those hearty enough to swim in cold Lake Ontario, men's and women's change rooms were located inside the impressive-looking bathing pavilion, which still stands on the south side of the Lake Shore Boulevard. It was modeled after a similar-looking though much smaller bathing pavilion in Lynn Beach, Massachusetts. The cold lake water became too much and a huge, new swimming pool was built just to the east of the bathing pavilion in 1925 (see 124). The number of visitors to Sunnyside peaked during the war years then slowly dropped off. By the early 1950s, the car had become king and fewer and fewer people frequented Sunnyside. The park, rides, and restaurants grew tackier and tackier and, following the 1955 season and several suspicious fires, Sunnyside Amusement Park closed. Most of the rides were quickly dismantled and the rest of the park flattened in early 1956 during the construction of the Gardiner Expressway. Today, except for a precious few landmarks like the bathing pavilion, pool, and Palais Royale dance hall, Toronto's Sunnyside Amusement Park is only a happy memory. An interesting feature of today's Sunnyside is that while the boardwalk remains, the original wood has been replaced using a material called Trex, a wood-like product made from recycled plastic garbage bags.

\* \* \* \* \*

TORONTO TRANSIT COMMISSION'S RONCESVALLES CARHOUSE (121): High on the embankment to the north is one of the two remaining TTC carhouses. Four years after the Toronto Railway Company was established in 1891 to look after the city's public transportation needs, a carhouse was built just north of the complicated and busy intersection of King Street, Queen Street, Roncesvalles Avenue, The Queensway, and (until 1956) Lakeshore Road. In the early years of this century, more than two hundred streetcars were stored in and around the carhouse until a larger, more modem structure became necessary. The new building, which can be seen high on the embankment overlooking Sunnyside, was erected by the newly formed Toronto Transportation Commission (since 1954, Toronto Transit Commission) in 1923 and is still in service as one of Toronto's two operating streetcar divisions, the other being Russell Division on Queen Street East. Today, more than 150 streetcars operating on the Queen, King, Dundas, Carlton, Bathurst, and St. Clair routes are serviced and stored at the TTC's Roncesvalles carhouse. Next door is St. Joe's Hospital.

ST. JOSEPH'S HEALTH CENTRE, 30 The Queensway (122): The Congregation of the Sisters of St. Joseph, which was established in Le Puy, France, in 1648, had its Toronto beginnings in 1851 when four sisters who had been overseeing an orphanage in Philadelphia arrived in our city to take charge of a similar, but much smaller institution on Nelson Street (the former name of that part of Jarvis Street south of Queen). In 1859, the children from the Nelson Street orphanage were moved to the new House of Providence on Power Street where they were looked after until 1876. Then, in that year, the sisters acquired a beautiful piece of property overlooking the lake just west of the Town of Parkdale. In 1885, the sisters bought the property, added a wing to the existing structure and renamed their institution Sacred Heart Orphanage. In the early summer of 1921, the sisters got word that their buildings were going to be expropriated and demolished by the city in order that a new high school could be built. The sisters did some quick thinking and by October, 1921, the last of the orphans had been moved to other facilities and the first patient had been admitted to the sister's new St. Joseph's Hospital. The law said that a hospital could not be expropriated. Since then, a much remodelled "St. Joe's" has grown to become one of Toronto's busiest and most respected health care facilities.

\* \* \* \* \*

## Continue west along Lake Shore Boulevard

BUDAPEST PARK (123): This city park was established by act of city council on June 22 of 1966 to commemorate the tenth anniversary of the Hungarian Revolution.

PARKSIDE DRIVE: Until April 11, 1921, Parkside Drive was simply a southerly extension of Keele Street. On that date, city council approved a name change for the lower part of Keele to Parkside Drive as requested by local residents. The residents felt the new name was better from a real estate point of view than the more industrial sounding Keele Street. Thus, since that April date, the name Keele has been used only for that portion of the thoroughfare above Bloor Street running north past the Union Stock Yards and abattoirs to St. Clair Avenue. A brief aside ... Keele Street was named for William Keele, a lawyer who owned land adjacent to the thoroughfare that took his name. He also owned the Carlton Race Course southwest of the Keele and Dundas Street intersection where the first Queen's Plate was held in 1860. Incidentally, the park Parkside is at the side of is High Park, a major portion of which was granted to the city by its owner, John George Howard.

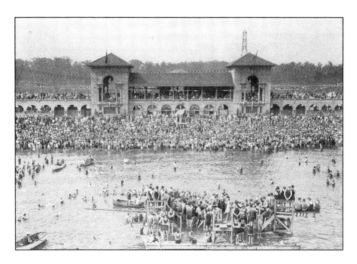

Thousands flocked to the Water Nymph Carnival at the Sunnyside Bathing pavilion, 1923.

GUS RYDER SUNNYSIDE POOL (124): In 1925, to overcome the problem of having to swim in a cold Lake Ontario, a new $75,000 swimming "tank" (a term unique to the locals) opened. This tank, or pool, could accommodate two thousand swimmers at one time, each of whom would have paid an admission fee of thirty-five cents (ten cents for children). In 1963, admission fees were abolished and in 1985, the tank's name was changed to the Gus Ryder Sunnyside Pool. Gus, a prominent swimming coach whose most famous pupil was Marilyn Bell (see 109), taught many of his young students in this pool, oops ... tank.

Construction of the SUNNYSIDE BATHING PAVILION (125), located on the south side of Lake Shore Boulevard just west of the Sunnyside Gus Ryder Pool, was started in 1921 and completed the following year in time for the opening of the park on June 18. Built by the owners of the park, the Toronto Harbour Commission, the pseudoclassical structure was designed by Toronto architect Alfred Chapman, who was also responsible for the Toronto Harbour Commission Building at 60 Harbour Street (see 33) and the Princes' Gates at the CNE grounds (see 84). Large enough to provide changing facilities for some 7,700 bathers at one time (men and women on separate sides, of course), the handsome structure was based on a similar, though much smaller bathing pavilion at Lynn Beach, Massachusetts. In recent years more than $1 million has been spent by the city to help preserve this landmark of a by-gone era. During the warmer months a fashionable restaurant welcomes visitors to the pavilion.

COLBORNE LODGE DRIVE: This thoroughfare leads into (and out of) High Park, the city's second largest public park (Toronto Island is the largest) which is located north of Lake Shore Boulevard, the Gardiner Expressway, railway tracks, and The Queensway. Now encompassing 398 acres (161 hectares), the original 165-acre (66-hectare) portion of High Park was bequeathed to the city by its owner John George Howard in 1873 on the condition that the city provided Howard and his wife a yearly annuity of $1,200. The city fathers almost declined the offer because, as one said, the property was too far out in the country. Howard's 165-acre "gift" ultimately cost the city almost $20,000.

Howard called his residence, which he built in 1837 at the south end of his property overlooking the lake, COLBORNE LODGE (126) after his good friend and mentor Sir John Colborne, the founder of Upper Canada College who gave the position of drawing master in the new school to Howard. Colborne also served as Upper Canada's seventh lieutenant-governor from 1828–1836.

SIR CASIMIR GZOWSKI PARK (127): Gzowski was born in St. Petersburg, Russia in 1813 of Polish parents. In 1831, following an unsuccessful insurrection by the Polish military and citizenry against the Russians, Gzowski, who had been studying military engineering, fled to France then across the Atlantic to the "New World." To help him learn the English language, Gzowski practiced law and passed his bar examinations in 1837. His preference, however, was for engineering and in 1841 he moved to Canada where he obtained, through his friendship with Governor General Sir Charles Bagot, a position with the Federal Department of Public Works. The railway boom was just starting in Canada and, recognizing its bright future, Gzowski was appointed chief engineer of the proposed St. Lawrence and Sarnia Railroad. Four years later, Gzowski started his own construction firm and won the contract to build the Grand Trunk Railway's new line between Toronto and Sarnia, which he completed in 1857. To make the high quality rails for the project, he and his partners founded the Toronto Rolling Mills, the first factory in Canada to manufacture iron rails. Another of Gzowski's major achievements was the construction of the International Bridge across the Niagara River between Buffalo and Fort Erie. Of particular interest to students of Toronto's waterfront history was Gzowski's 1853 plan for a cross-waterfront esplanade that would provide an elevated access for the Grand Trunk Railway's new tracks from Montreal into the city in conjunction with a tree-lined recreation and pleasure ground for the citizens. Work started on the project, but with a change in the civic administration prior to it's completion, Gzowski's contract was cancelled.

Almost thirty-five years later, the railways owned virtually all of Toronto's waterfront. Gzowski, who had taken up residence in a large house near the corner of Bathurst and Dundas Streets, was again asked to offer assistance to help salvage some of the city's new waterfront for the citizens. Again he made a plea to reserve a portion of the land that was in the process of being reclaimed for the citizens and again the politicians failed to listen. It's interesting to speculate what Toronto's waterfront might be like if Gzowski's ideas had been heeded. In 1890, this distinguished Canadian was knighted by Queen Victoria for his many civic and military services. The Gzowski Memorial in this park was designed by Polish-Canadian architect Richard D'Wonnik and was unveiled by Prime Minister Pierre Trudeau on May 25, 1968. The three sets of railway tracks leading to and from the centre of the memorial are from a portion of the original Grand Trunk line from Toronto to Sarnia laid down by Gzowski during the period 1853–1857. The bare girders protruding from the top of the memorial symbolize the belief that an engineer's work is never complete.

\*   \*   \*   \*   \*

ELLIS AVENUE: This street is named for John Ellis Sr., who arrived in Toronto from England and was convinced by his neighbour John George Howard of High Park to purchase what is now Grenadier Pond and the 165 acres (66 hectares) to the west of the pond for $25 an acre. In 1839, Ellis built for himself a house near the foot of today's Ellis Avenue, a house he called Herne Hill after his home in England.

INN ON THE LAKE, 1926 Lake Shore Boulevard West (128): During the 1940s, Lou Epstein opened his Downyflake doughnut shop ("As you go through life, brother, what ever be your goal, keep your eye upon the doughnut, and not upon the hole") in the heart of the Sunnyside Amusement Park. A few years later he built the Sunnyside Motel on the north side of Lake Shore Boulevard just east of the Humber River traffic bridge. In 1952, he tore the scruffy little motel down and built the 155-room Seaway Motel which, in 1984, was renamed the Inn On The Lake.

WINDERMERE AVENUE: The post office that served the little community that had developed in the late 1800s near the foot of today's Windermere Avenue at the old Lakeshore Road was originally named Windermere Post Office by John Ellis's son John Jr. after Lake Windermere, the largest freshwater lake in England, Ellis's homeland. Because it was frequently confused with an existing Windermere Post Office in Muskoka, the name was changed in 1890 to Swansea after Swansea in Wales, both communities having extensive steel works and rolling mills. On January 1, 1967, the Village of Swansea joined the City of Toronto becoming part of Ward 7.

OLCO GASOLINE STATION, 1978 Lake Shore Boulevard West (129): This unique little structure is the last of its kind still standing in our city. It was built in 1937 by the Hercules Oil Company of Detroit, Michigan, a company that, following the death of its owner Herbert Austin, was renamed the Joy Oil Company by his widow. At one time there was a total of sixteen similar-looking Joy gasoline stations scattered around Toronto. The "chateau" style of architecture is reminiscent of a time when motoring was a romantic adventure, not a tiresome task. Following Joy Oil Company's departure from the Canadian scene the stations were operated by a succession of independent operators.

QUEEN ELIZABETH WAY (QEW) MONUMENT (130): When the QEW was officially opened at the Henley Bridge in St. Catharines in June of 1939 by King George VI and Queen Elizabeth, it was the longest divided highway in the world. Actually, the idea for a new traffic artery between Toronto and the Niagara Peninsula originated as far back as 1931.

The new highway would utilize an existing two-lane thoroughfare called the Middle Road (since it was located between Lakeshore Road and Dundas Street) that would be widened to 40 feet (12 metres) and incorporate four lanes of traffic, two in each direction separated by a centre boulevard. At the time this was a revolutionary concept in highway design. The first section of this new highway between Niagara Falls and Highway 27 (now Highway 427), on the western outskirts of Toronto, opened in 1939 and the stretch between Highway 27 and the entrance to Toronto at the Humber River in the summer of 1940. The graceful, impressive Queen Elizabeth Way monument (which was relocated to a small park south of Lake Shore Boulevard and away from the traffic in 1974) originally stood at the city end of the bridge between the east and westbound traffic lanes over the Humber River. It was erected in 1939 to commemorate the arrival of the new highway at Toronto's doorstep. The snarling eight-foot-high stone lion was sculpted by Toronto's Frances Loring and represents a "defiant British lion" on guard for England during the early part of the Second World War. Coincident with the creation of the new City of Toronto on January 1, 1998, the section of the provincially maintained QEW from the Humber River to the old Metro Toronto boundary at Etobicoke Creek became part of the Gardiner Expressway and is now under the jurisdiction of the city.

The HUMBER RIVER, which forms Toronto's westerly boundary with the former City of Etobicoke (a name that means "where the black alders trees grow" in Ojibway), was named by Elizabeth Simcoe, wife of Toronto's founder John Graves Simcoe, after the Humber River in the northeast of England. Into this English river flows the Don, the name of our city's other major watercourse that empties into Toronto Bay at the east end of the harbour. It too was named by Mrs. Simcoe in recognition of the Don River in Yorkshire, England. For hundreds of years, Humber was used by Indians and explorers as a portage route from the north country to Lake Ontario. The first white person to view the future site of Toronto, explorer Samuel Champlain's guide Étienne Brûlé, travelled down the "Toronto passage," as the Humber River was also known, in 1615.

The HUMBER RIVER PEDESTRIAN AND BICYCLE BRIDGE (131): There have been many bridges constructed over the mouth of the Humber River. The first one, erected in the early 1800s, carried the York-Niagara stagecoaches, riders on horseback, and wagons headed to or from the St. Lawrence Market. It was replaced by ever-more substantial structures, but none were as spectacular as this bridge which soars five storeys into the air and was opened to the public in late 1994. Note particularly the thunderbirds that help brace the twin 4-foot (1.2-metre) diameter pipeline steel arches while carved turtles and serpents guide the

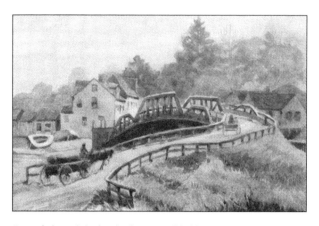

One of the original Lakeshore Road bridges across the Humber River, circa 1840.

way. The bridge was assembled on the east bank of the river. The arches, with deck suspended beneath, were floated into position using barges to cross the river mouth. The arch span is 328 feet (100 metres), the bridge 456 feet (139.2 metres) in total length and the top of arch is 81 feet (24.8 metres) over the water. The reinforced deck slab was cast on steel cross-beams and is suspended from the arches by forty-four stainless steel rods. To the north of this bridge are more utilitarian bridges that carry the many lanes of the busy Gardiner Expressway over the river. The replacement of the six bridges will necessitate more than $100-million worth of construction over the next several years.

Site of the PALACE PIER (132): The names of these two condominiums reflect the fact that they were constructed on and near the site of one of the city's most popular dance halls, the Palace Pier. As first proposed the structure was to be a half-mile long amusement pier similar to many found in England. It was, in fact, named for Brighton's Palace Pier. Unfortunately, things didn't quite work out and all that was actually constructed was a 300-foot-long (914 metres) structure that opened as a roller skating rink in 1931. Over the years, the Palace Pier hosted wrestling, boxing matches, and religious revival meetings, but is best remembered as an extremely popular dance hall. The building was totally destroyed by an arsonist on January 7, 1963. A portion of a pier footing, to which a descriptive plaque is attached, can be seen at the south end of nearby Palace Pier Court.

## End of Walk One

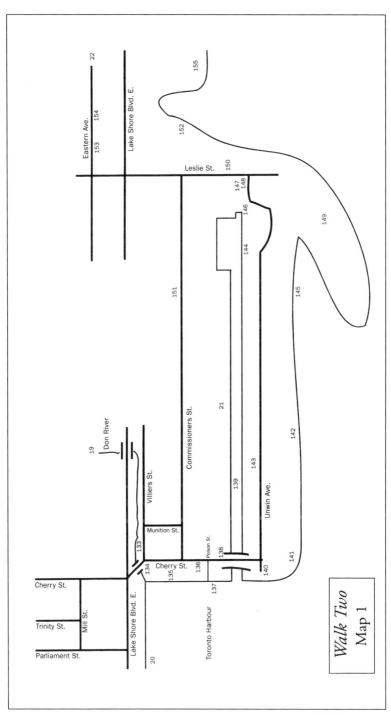

Eastern Ave.

Lake Shore Blvd. E.

22

153  154

155

152

Leslie St.

150

147
148

146

149

144

151

21

145

Don River

19

Villiers St.

Commissioners St.

139

143

Unwin Ave.

142

Munition St.

133

Poison St.

138

140

141

134

Cherry St.

135

136

Cherry St.

Mill St.

137

Trinity St.

Toronto Harbour

Lake Shore Blvd. E.

Parliament St.

20

*Walk Two*
Map 1

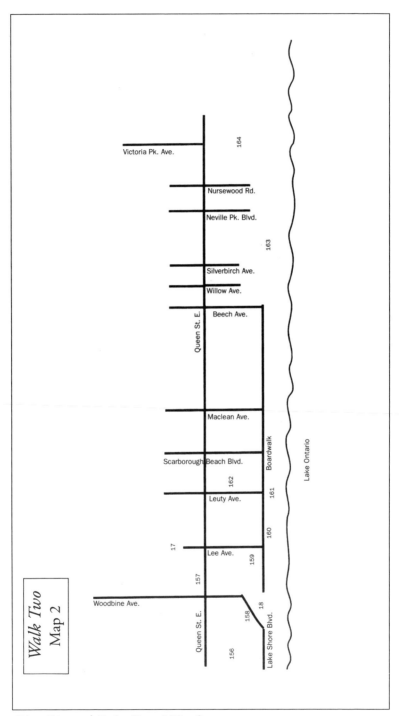

Walk Two
Map 2

Victoria Pk. Ave.

164

Nursewood Rd.

Neville Pk. Blvd.

163

Silverbirch Ave.

Willow Ave.

Queen St. E.

Beech Ave.

Maclean Ave.

Boardwalk

Lake Ontario

Scarborough Beach Blvd.

162

161

Leuty Ave.

160

17

Lee Ave.

159

157

Woodbine Ave.

158

18

Queen St. E.

Lake Shore Blvd.

156

# Walk Two

## Port Lands to the R.C. Harris
## Water Treatment Plant

The second walk in our trio of walks begins just south of the Gooderham and Worts complex where Walk One began.

**Walk begins on Cherry Street**
**just south of Lake Shore Boulevard**

**Proceed south on Cherry Street**

The area we are entering originally formed the east "wall" of Toronto Bay and was referred to, at the time of its creation by the Toronto Harbour Commission earlier this century, as the Toronto Eastern Harbour Terminals District. In our city's formative years this area was nothing more than acres and acres of boggy marshes known as Ashbridge's Bay after the Ashbridge family that settled in the early 1800s out in the countryside near the intersection of today's Queen Street East and Greenwood Avenue. Part of the Toronto Harbour Commission's massive $19-million waterfront redevelopment plan (which received final approval by city council in 1912) was a proposal to create hundreds of acres of useable land by filling in Ashbridge's Bay with dredgings from Toronto Bay. A new, more direct channel for the murky, slow-moving Don River to follow on its way to Toronto Bay as well as a 6,800-foot-long (2,073 metres) ship channel with 3 miles (4.8 kilometres) of dockage along its concrete walls and a large turning basin at its east end were also to be included in the project. The channel was subsequently named in honour of Edward H. Keating, the city engineer from 1892 to 1898. The City of Toronto Handbook for the year 1917 predicted there would one day be one thousand factories established in the new Eastern Harbour Terminal district. Work started on this phase of the THC's waterfront redevelopment plan in 1914 and within four years, more than 74 acres (30 hectares) of new land had been created through the almost continuous use of Cyclone, the largest and most powerful floating dredge on the continent. By 1922, another 432 acres (175 hectares) had been reclaimed and 5.6 miles (9 kilometres) of watermains, 2.4 miles (3.9 kilometres) of storms sewers and 10.3 miles (16.6 kilometres) of railway sidings were in place. Work continued at a brisk pace. As new land was reclaimed and serviced, all manner of industries moved in, the first being the British Forgings Limited plant where scrap steel from across Canada was melted using an electric current and processed into steel forgings and shells for the war effort. This plant was erected in the incredibly short period of less than seven months, and eventually covered 127 acres (51.8 hectares) of newly reclaimed land and employed 1,600 workers (who got to and from work on the short-lived Ashbridge streetcar route that connected with the Queen line). At the time it was the largest electric steel factory in the world. By war's end the plant had turned out 48,000 tons of steel and more than three million shells. We are reminded of this once-important harbour industry through the name of a nearby thoroughfare, Munitions Street. By 1931, forty-one industries ranging from oil refiners and coal storage yards to light and heavy manufacturing operations had settled in Toronto's new Eastern Harbour Terminal. In the pre-fuel oil and electric heat days, coal was a major commodity passing through the new terminal district with more than a million tons from mines in Canada, the United States, Wales, and Scotland off-loaded in 1932 to eventually be sold by sixteen major Toronto coal dealers to an eager, and shivering, populace. Over the next two decades, the pace of development work in the Eastern Harbour Terminal district slackened. Then, in the early 1950s, anticipating increased activity in the Port of Toronto with the completion of the new St. Lawrence Seaway, the Harbour Commission began developing new plans for the east end of Toronto Harbour. In recent years much of the heavy industry scattered throughout the area began moving out, leaving the once-busy terminal district with serious problems. A Royal Commission on the Future of the Toronto Waterfront was established to look at the situation. Following the release of its 1990 report, ownership of some 400+ acres (160+ hectares) of land in the Port Area was transferred to the Toronto Economic Development Corporation (TEDCO), which had been established by the city in 1986 as the more appropriate agency to look at ways and means of revitalizing those lands along Queen's Quay East and in the Port Area (formerly the Eastern Harbour Terminal District). Other private sector proposals for the Port Lands include a three-pad hockey and skating arena, several warehouse-style retail outlet stores, and a number of warehouses, offices, and industrial buildings. There is also a possibility that much of the property on the west side of Cherry Street between the Keating Channel and Polson Street will be utilized as the site of the Olympic Village should Toronto be awarded the 2008 Summer Games. Venues for the various sporting events are also planned all along the waterfront with special emphasis placed on Exhibition Place, Ontario Place, SkyDome, and the new Air Canada Centre.

VILLIERS STREET, just north of Commissioners Street, was named for Matthew Villiers Sankey, the city surveyor from 1888 to 1905. Shortly after retiring from the public service, Sankey was drowned in a boating accident near Kenora, Ontario.

THE IRISH ROVERS PUB (133) opened in 1996 and is one of the amenities that's been added to the area to serve the residents of this evolving "business park" located just minutes from downtown Toronto.

ESSROC CANADA (134) operates the huge silo on the west side of Cherry Street just south of the bridge. Here shipments of cement that arrive from Picton, Ontario, are stored prior to distribution by truck throughout this part of the province. Frequently seen unloading at the nearby dock is the *Stephen B. Roman* (formerly the *Fort William*).

MARINE TERMINAL 35 (135) was built in the early 1960s on the site of the once-busy coal storage yards of the Canada Coal and Elias Rogers Coal companies. This terminal has 140,000 square feet (13,000 square metres) of inside storage space with an additional 23.3 acres (9.3 hectares) outside. These combined areas are known collectively as the E.L. Cousins Docks, named in honour of the THC's first chief engineer and general manager.

Towering over the Docks is the Toronto Harbour Commission's huge 300-ton (272-tonne) capacity ATLAS CRANE (136), which was first used in 1962.

COMMISSIONERS STREET intersects Cherry Street opposite the E.L. Cousins Docks and was named for the first five gentlemen to be appointed as Toronto Harbour Commissioners in 1911; Messrs. L.H. Clarke (Chairman), T.L. Church, R.S. Gourlay, R. Home Smith, and F.S. Spence.

\* \* \* \* \*

POLSON STREET was formerly known as Carton Street after the Dominion Boxboard Company's carton factory that was located on the south side of the street. The present name commemorates a former harbour industry, the Polson Iron Works Company, which was established in 1883 at the foot of Princess Street on the old waterfront by William Polson. Polson's was an extremely active shipbuilding yard where hundreds of vessels, including the Island ferry *Trillium* and RCYC private launch *Kwasind*, were launched. This once-prosperous company went bankrupt in 1919 thanks in great measure to the indifference of the federal government then in power.

THE DOCKS ENTERTAINMENT COMPLEX (137) at the west end Polson Street is a new entertainment complex that opened in 1996 and features a casual restaurant, swinging nightclub, a 41,000-square-foot lakeside licenced patio, and several outdoor sports venues including swimming pool, beach volleyball courts and an 18-hole professional mini-putt golf course.

Technically known as the CHERRY STREET STRAUSS TRUNNION BASCULE BRIDGE (138) this is one of two bridges on Cherry Street. It was built by the Strauss Engineering Corporation, Chicago and the Dominion Bridge Company, Montreal and opened to traffic on June 29, 1931. The massive bridge counterweights consist of 750 tons (680.6 tonnes) of concrete. The use of relatively inexpensive concrete in place of costly iron for bascule bridge counterweights was a feature patented by the Strauss Company, an enterprise founded by Joseph Baermann Strauss, the same man who built the famous $35-million Golden Gate Bridge in San Francisco, which took four years to construct and opened on May 27, 1937.

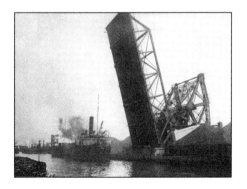

Cherry Street bascule bridge, 1931

The SHIP CHANNEL (139) was built as an integral part of the Eastern Harbour Terminal project. It runs east from Toronto Bay into the heart of the terminal and is 6,800 feet (2,073 metres) in length, 400 feet (122 metres) wide and 24 feet (7.3 metres) deep. The Ship Channel terminates in a turning basin 1,100 feet (335 metres) square. Adjacent to the channel are mountains of road salt. More than 400,000 tonnes arrive annually.

MARINE TERMINAL 51 and the CONTAINER DISTRIBUTION CENTRE COMPLEX (140): Just west of the Cherry Street-Unwin Avenue intersection is Marine Terminal 51, which was built in 1966 at a cost of $2 million. This sprawling complex includes a 150,000 square feet (13,935 square metres) of inside storage space with an additional 19 acres (7.6 hectares) outside storage. Adjacent is the Container Distribution Centre, a 25-acre (10-hectare) complex that includes a 100,000-square-foot (9,290-square-metre) warehouse. The facility offers importer and exporter alike complete packing, unpacking, distribution, and bonded storage areas with easy access to trans-shipment by rail or highway transportation modes. The centre is a "RO-RO" facility where wheeled cargoes and containers on chassis as well as heavy equipment can be RO-lled on or RO-lled off ships. Just north of the security gate controlling entry to this property is the Missions to Seamen, better known as the Flying Angel, a popular gathering place for visiting sailors. One of the buildings used by the mission is a former TTC Peter Witt trailer. Now painted blue, it was one of 225 similar cars that along with their electrified companions, the Witt "motors," transported hundreds of thousands of Torontonians to and from work and play during the 1920s into the early 1960s.

CHERRY BEACH (141): Also known as Clarke Beach after Alderman Harry Clarke who, in 1932, did much to have such public amenities as a concession stand and change rooms built for those seeking a cool (actually chilly) dip in Lake Ontario.

UNWIN AVENUE was named for Charles Unwin, a pioneer provincial land surveyor (he had certificate #17) and a member of the surveying company Wadsworth, Unwin and Brown that surveyed Toronto Island soon after the former peninsula was severed from the mainland in 1858.

## Proceed east along Unwin Avenue

FISHERMAN'S ISLAND and SIMCOE PARK (site of, 142): Proceeding east along Unwin Avenue we are actually traversing what was a long, narrow peninsula separated from the city to the north by the marshes and swamps of an extended Ashbridge's Bay. A community of fishermen (thus the name) took up residence in a collection of shanties fabricated from the flotsam and jetsam washed ashore from the lake. At its peak, thirty families resided on Fisherman's Island until the land reclamation program instigated by the Toronto Harbour Commission forced them to move. By the early 1920s, this part of the sandbar was vacant. Simcoe Park, at the east end of Fisherman's Island, had been developed as a public park in 1906. It attained a peak summertime population of two hundred before it too was cleared so that landfilling could begin. Between the park and Fisherman's Island was a small Anglican church, St. Nicholas, which served the community's needs until it was demolished in 1921. All the industries now found along Unwin Avenue sit on land reclaimed by the commission as it created the new Eastern Harbour Terminals District.

STRADA HARBOUR AGGREGATES (143): This company, which opened on this site in early 1996, is in the recycling business — though in a rather unique way. When the city undertakes a major road rebuilding project, the concrete base (not the asphalt) is trucked to this plant where it is converted into various sizes of crushed aggregate and subsequently reused in other construction projects. This type of industry fulfils TEDCO's desire to retain part of the Port Lands for various recycling plants.

RICHARD L. HEARN GENERATING STATION (144): This plant, which was built soon after the end of the Second World War to help alleviate

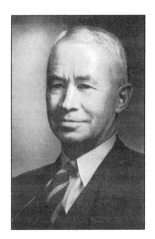

Richard L. Hearn

a critical power shortage throughout the province, was named in honour of Ontario Hydro's seventh chairman, a position Richard Lankaster Hearn held from January, 1955, until his retirement in October of the following year. Hearn replaced Robert Hood Saunders (a former Toronto mayor) who had been killed in a plane crash at the London, Ontario airport. Hearn had joined Hydro following graduation from the University of Toronto in 1913, just seven years after the commission was established. Over the years Hearn held several important positions with Ontario Hydro and with other energy companies. He was also involved with the development of the Candu nuclear program and the creation of Atomic Energy of Canada. When asked about the renaming of this power station in his honour (it had been erected in the early 1950s as the Scarborough Generating Station) Hearn commented, "here they are naming a steam plant after me and I don't know anything about steam! Nothing at all!" Though built as a coal-fired station, increasing community concerns about air quality resulted in the conversion of the plant to natural gas and in 1971 the construction of the mammoth chimney to better disperse stack gases. Soon a surplus of electrical generating capacity throughout the province combined with an ever-increasing number of plant operating inefficiencies resulted in the facility, the largest thermal (steam) generating station in the country when it opened in 1951, to be gradually taken "off line." The last of the eight units was shut down in the summer of 1983. Recently, there has been talk of constructing a technologically up-to-date gas-fired station on the property to take advantage of the network of electrical switching gears seen north of the plant and adjacent to the Ship Channel. Hearn died on May 26, 1987 at the age of 95.

OUTER HARBOUR MARINA (145): Set in a park-like setting and operated by the Toronto Harbour Commission, this facility has slips to accommodate up to 654 craft, sail or power, plus such amenities as power, fuel, washrooms, showers, etc.

TORONTO DRYDOCK (146): In 1983 this unique ship, the former Great Lakes pulp carrier *Menier Consol*, was converted into a floating drydock. Vessels, to a maximum 40 feet (12.2 metres) in width and 200 feet (61 metres) in length, are floated into the drydock, which is full of water. The water is then pumped out, leaving the vessel high and dry. Necessary inspections and repairs are then undertaken.

STAR CHOICE NETWORK, INC. (147): This facility is used by the company as a broadcast centre for its "direct-to-home" television operations.

TELESAT CANADA COMMUNICATIONS INC. (148): Telesat Canada was established in 1969 to provide telecommunications services. Its Teleport Toronto satellite transmission station was established here in 1986 and serves customers from coast to coast via its myriad of antennas.

LESLIE STREET is named for George Leslie, who ran a nursery not far from the present Queen and Leslie intersection. The community that developed nearby became known as Leslieville and the north-south Second Concession Road, which was laid out by the surveyors exactly 2 1/2 miles east of Yonge Street (one concession = 6,600 feet = 1 1/4 miles), naturally took on the name of the area's most prominent citizen. It is said that George Leslie gave his friend Alexander Muir the title of the song the latter was to enter in a patriotic song contest being held in Montreal. Having written the melody, Muir needed a title and when Leslie noticed that a leaf from a maple tree had fallen and clung to his friend's coat sleeve, offered the words "The Maple Leaf Forever."

TOMMY THOMPSON PARK (149): At the south end of Leslie Street is what is known as the Leslie Street Spit, a land form originally created as a result of the dumping of inert materials removed from various construction sites around the city. The new Leslie Street Spit was to form a breakwall to protect the new Outer Harbour which, in turn, was to replace the wharves and docking facilities along the Inner Harbour. This plan never materialized and natural regeneration of the Spit soon began to take place. The park is named for the late Tommy Thompson, who was Metropolitan Toronto's first parks commissioner, a position he held for more than twenty years. It was Tommy who gave us the "Please Walk on the Grass" signs.

## Proceed north on Leslie Street

LESLIE STREET ALLOTMENT GARDENS (150): These small plots, which rent for twenty dollars a season, have been under cultivation for more than twenty years. They afford a place for people who live in apartments or those in houses without gardens to get their knees dirty. Here on Leslie Street there are approximately 235 plots each measuring 10 feet (3 metres) by 20 feet (6 metres). As one would imagine, there is a substantial waiting list to obtain a plot.

TORONTO HYDRO SERVICE CENTRE (151): A short detour west off Leslie Street to 500 Commissioners Street takes us to Toronto Hydro's new Service Centre, a 650,000-square-foot facility that brings together all the service, construction, maintenance, trades training, and materials management functions of the utility on one site. This project, which was fully operational on March 1, 1997, is the first of the newcomers to the TEDCO-managed Port Lands. Toronto Hydro's arrival gives an indication of the future uses awaiting this once-depressed area.

## Proceed east on Lake Shore Boulveard

MAIN SEWAGE TREATMENT PLANT (152): As we turn the corner and proceed east on Lake Shore Boulevard on the south side of the street we can see the sprawling Main Sewage Treatment Plant. Covering more than forty hectares it is the largest water pollution control plant in the city. Construction of the first treatment plant on this site began in 1910 when the city's population was slightly less than 350,000. Since then the facility has been constantly upgraded with the first components of the present plant erected in 1943. In the intervening years various additions have been made that now allow complete waste water treatment to take place, i.e. primary sedimentation followed by aeration followed by final sedimentation. The raw influent arrives from various parts of the city via six enormous sewers and following treatment the effluent is chlorinated and discharged into the lake through a series of eight diffusers approximately 1,000 metres (3,280 feet) offshore. The plant now serves 1.5 million residents and treats an average daily flow of approximately 800,000 cubic metres. To meet ever-tightening waste water criteria additional upgrades are planned.

TORONTO FIRE ACADEMY (153): On the north side of Lake Shore Boulevard we can see part of the Toronto Fire Academy, its presence made obvious by the blackened railway tank car and house-like structure, both of which are part of the academy's training apparatus. Before this facility opened training took place using a brick drill tower behind the old No. 1 hall on Adelaide Street east of University Avenue, and later at No. 23 Fire Station on Howland Avenue. The modern Toronto Fire Academy on Eastern Avenue was officially opened on October 9, 1970. At one time a fire museum was located in the academy. It's anticipated that the artifacts will become part of the new Harbourfront Fire Hall on Queen's Quay West (see 44).

CANADA POST SOUTH CENTRAL LETTER PROCESSING PLANT (154): With its main entrance on Eastern Avenue this facility, which opened in 1975, processes, on average, more than 5 million letters a day. This volume makes this South Central the largest letter sorting plant in the country.

ASHBRIDGE'S BAY PARK — WOODBINE BEACH (155): Located here are the Toronto Beaches Lion's Jonathan Ashbridge Community Centre, the Toronto Hydroplane and Sailing Club and the Ashbridge's Bay Yacht Club. The latter was established in this general vicinity in 1932 in the pre-manicured days of the present park. The club met in three different locations with the present site opening in 1977. Total membership is about 450 and the club fleet approximates 250 craft of all sizes. This park and the adjacent Woodbine Beach are popular places for family picnics and outings.

COXWELL AVENUE was named for Charles Coxwell Small, a pioneer neighbourhood property owner who held 472 acres (189 hectares) in an area now bounded by the lakefront, Woodbine, Danforth, and Coxwell avenues. Small was born in York (Toronto) in 1800 and at the age of 25 succeeded his father as Clerk of the Crown and Pleas. Small also served as colonel of the 4th York Militia. He died in 1864. A small pond on his property took the name Small's Pond.

WOODBINE RACE TRACK, renamed OLD WOODBINE, then GREENWOOD (site of, 156): Horse racing has always been a popular sport in Toronto and when the Woodbine trotting and running track opened in 1875 it was added to a list that already included Charlie Keele's Carelton chase course in northwest Toronto, Maitland's track ("south of Queen Street over the Don"), Gate's Newmarket course (east of the city near today's Danforth Avenue and Main Street), and Scarlett's Simcoe race course close to where Dundas Street crossed the Humber River. The first in that list was the city's pioneer track across the bay on the peninsula (Toronto Island). The list would be extended to include such future tracks as Thorncliffe, Long Branch, Dufferin, and a new Woodbine in north Etobicoke near the Toronto airport. All have vanished, save for the last mentioned. The original Woodbine Riding and Driving Park was named for the Woodbine Hotel at 88 Yonge Street. Pardee and Howell, owners of the Woodbine hotel, purchased the Queen Street East property from Joe Duggan in 1874. Not an instant hit, the course's proximity to the waterfront led to flooding problems that required frequent repair work to be done to the dirt track. Nevertheless, it was decided to hold the seventeenth running of the coveted Queen's Plate at the track, which now had the simplified title of Woodbine Park, on May 31, 1876. This was a week later than planned due to, what else, a flooded track. If it ever comes up on the TV game show "Jeopardy," the winning mount that year was Norah P. Exactly eighty years later the running of the Queen's Plate was moved to the New Woodbine and the Queen Street track was renamed Old Woodbine. Another piece of trivia — the last Queen's Plate winner at the original Woodbine track was Ace Marine. Over the next few years Old Woodbine saw hundreds of harness races both under that name and, after 1963, Greenwood. All horse racing at the historic track ended on December 31, 1993. Redevelopment of the site was first announced a year later, but soon controversy clouded future uses of the 81-acre (33-hectare) site. Present plans (1998) call for almost nine hundred new housing units made up of semi-detached and fully detached houses, townhouses, and condominiums, the latter type to be built along the Queen Street frontage. The houses will line the newly laid out streets at the east end of the property. The streets have been given the names Boardwalk (in recognition of the popular Eastern Beaches Park boardwalk), Sara Ashbridge (pioneer area settler), Smalls Corners (the name of the small community that evolved at the Queen Street/Kingston Road intersection, see COXWELL AVENUE), Glenn Gould (the world renowned Toronto-born pianist and one-time area resident), Northern Dancer, to honour the famous Canadian-bred race horse who won the Triple Crown of racing in 1964, and Joseph Duggan, in recognition of the site's original landowner. The condominiums will be located along the Queen Street frontage. There will also be a park, school, and sports facilities.

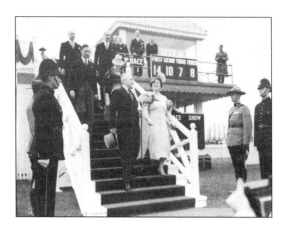

King George VI and Queen Elizabeth during their visit to Woodbine, 1939.

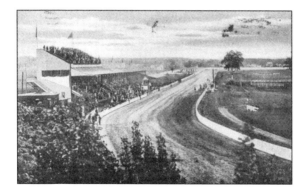

An old postcard view of Woodbine, 1914.

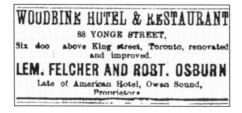

The track was named after the Woodbine Hotel on Yonge Street — 1881 newspaper ad.

TORONTO FIRE DEPARTMENT #17 FIRE HALL (157): Just visible north and east of the former race track site, east of the Woodbine Avenue and Queen (Queen Victoria) Street intersection is the distinctive tower of the Toronto Fire Department's #17 Fire Hall. The Kew Beach community had been served by a volunteer fire brigade since the early 1890s. In 1904, members of this brigade rushed to the city's aid when the big fire of that year nearly destroyed all of downtown Toronto. In 1905–6, three years before what had become the Town of East Toronto was annexed by the big City of Toronto and perhaps in anticipation of this occurrence (or maybe because of the help the firefighters had given the city during the "Great Toronto Fire" of 1904), Toronto City Council authorized the construction of this fire hall, which at first housed a two-horse hose wagon and a city-paid crew consisting of a captain, lieutenant, driver, and a single fireman (though he may have been married — just a joke).

DONALD SUMMERVILLE OLYMPIC POOL (158): This Olympic-size swimming pool is dedicated to the memory of Don Summerville, a former mayor of Toronto who started his municipal political career in 1955 when he was elected an alderman for Ward 8, whose boundaries took in the site of this pool. His term in office as the city's chief magistrate was less than a year. Assuming office on January 1, 1963, Summerville suffered a fatal heart attack while playing in a benefit hockey game on November 19 of the same year. He was only the second mayor to die while in office. Sam McBride was the other (see Walk Three — Toronto Island ferry *Sam McBride*).

WOODBINE AVENUE was originally called the Third Concession Road east of Yonge Street since it was three concessions, or exactly 3 3/4 miles east of Yonge (each concession being 100 chains or 6,600 feet or 1 1/4 miles in width). The street was eventually given its present name because it led to and from the Woodbine Riding and Driving Track.

## Proceed east along the Boardwalk

THE BEACH DISTRICT has always had an identity crisis, at least as far as its name is concerned. The first settlers in the area, most of whom farmed the rich land referred to the area where they lived simply by the name of the closest beach — Woodbine, Kew, or Balmy. Kew is of particular interest because it was so named by Joseph Williams, an arrival from London, England, who settled in the area in 1853. In the summer of 1879, he opened a pleasure ground fronting on the lake which he referred to as "the Canadian Kew Gardens," an obvious reference to the beautiful Kew

Gardens or, to give the place its official title, the Royal Botanical Gardens which was established in the 18th century (or earlier) on the Thames River a few miles west of London. Soon the beach fronting this property took on the name, wait for it, Kew Beach. In 1907, the city purchased Williams' 20 acres (8 hectares) and this along with other adjacent properties was eventually merged into what is still known as Kew Gardens. Williams' c1902 house of stone at the foot of Lee Avenue (159) has been preserved as the parkkeeper's residence. As the small cottages and more substantial houses began to knit together and a community began to emerge, most of the locals began referring to the area as the Beach. Eventually, some of the new arrivals changed the name once again, this time pluralizing it to the Beaches. Which one's correct? To this day, the terms are used interchangeably, although most residents with a sense of community history still prefer to call it the Beach.

As mentioned, the first settlers in the area (the Ashbridges, the Smalls) eagerly farmed the land while later arrivals established their country residences here well away from the hustle and bustle of the busy City of Toronto far to the west. Several were to have their surnames applied to local streets that were cut through their respective properties, e.g. (Alfred Ernest) Ames and (Allan) MacLean (Howard). Then the entrepreneurs arrived and purchased large tracts of land, which were soon subdivided into building lots and sold off. Some of these people are recognized in the names of streets such as (Alex) Wheeler, (Walter Sutherland) Lee, and his wife, whose maiden name was (Emma Mary) Leuty. While all this activity was going on, the common folk from Toronto discovered the area and soon began journeying out to the Beach to find respite from the heat of the city by either sitting on the water's edge or visiting Victoria Park or Munro Park, each nestled amongst the forested meadows and each complete with benches, gentle rides, and refreshment booths. To assist with the visitor's trek out into the countryside, or the return trip back home, privately owned street railway companies laid track on Kingston Road and later along Queen Street, upon which their little cars would trundle having made connections with the big city streetcars. As the years went by, the Beach became more and more a part of the city, politically anyway, when the Town of East Toronto (which had come to include the Beach) was annexed by Toronto on December 15, 1908. Today they may be the same; nevertheless the Beach is different!

EASTERN BEACHES PARK (160): The opening of this park was described in the *Evening Telegram* newspaper as the "largest communal celebration in the history of any one section of the city." It was suggested that a joyful crowd of more than 50,000 was in attendance. One reason the May 24, 1932, event was so popular doubtlessly had to do with the length of time it took for the city to provide the Beach residents with their own neighbourhood park. A decade had passed since the people in west Toronto (in west Toronto!) got their park at Sunnyside, a fact the taxpayers in the Beach area just wouldn't let the politicians forget. Work on creating the new east end park finally got underway in late 1927 with the expropriation of a few rickety old cottages at Woodbine Beach at the west end of the park site while at the east end steps were taken to stop the serious erosion of sand through the building of groynes — small wooden jetties poking a dozen or so feet out into the lake. Work continued, albeit slowly since dozens of land and water lot claims had to be investigated. Nevertheless, more than two hundred houses and an uncounted number of boathouses all along the water's edge were eventually demolished thereby creating a long narrow grassy area north of a newly constructed boardwalk. On Victoria Day, 1932, the $2.4-million park (much of that money coming from appropriations put in place to help able-bodied victims of the Great Depression) was officially opened by Mayor William Stewart. The park came complete with the aforementioned 4,800-foot-long (1,463 metres) boardwalk (a portion of which has been replaced with Trex, a synthetic material made from recycled plastic garbage bags) and an athletic field, which was at first derisively referred to as Pantry Park since it was the size of a pantry. At the opening the mayor addressed the crowd briefly and then gave the signal for a Union Jack to be run up the flagpole while a band played "God Save the Queen," the national anthem of the day. Then, Miss Jessie Barchard, representing "the spirit of the Beaches," presented flowers to both Mrs. Stewart and Mrs. Chambers, wife of the Parks Commissioner, Charles E. Chambers. The celebration continued with a spectacular mile-long parade consisting of mounted policemen up front followed by bands, floats, costumed children, decorated automobiles, war veterans, and Scouts, that weaved its way up and down the streets of the community. The day continued with a series of sporting events, community dancing, open air moving pictures, and a concert by musicians of the 48th Highlanders, the Irish Regiment and the Kiwanis Boys Clubs Band. As dusk settled huge bonfires were lit and the jubilant spectators gathered round and lustily sang well into the night. Imagine, all this for a park. As things turned out the new park was a good news, bad news happening. The good news was that the community finally got its long-sought-after playground and the bad news was that a lot more people discovered the Beach. And they're still discovering it, hopefully with a copy of this guide in their hands.

LEUTY LIFE-SAVING STATION (161): Recently saved from demolition through a variety of citizen-inspired fund-raising projects, this little 1920 structure, which was designed by Alfred Chapman (of Princes' Gates and Ontario Government Building fame, see 84 and 108) seems to epitomize the grand old days when the entire community swam at the

Beach. Leuty Lifesaving Station restoration cost approximately $95,000, with fundraising covering about $38,000 of the total. The rest came from the city including a $5,000 grant from the Toronto Historical Board (now Heritage Toronto).

SCARBORO' BEACH AMUSEMENT PARK (site of, 162): Situated on the south side of Queen Street between the modern McLean and Leuty avenues, Scarboro' Beach Amusement Park opened for its first season on June 1, 1907. Covering almost 50 acres (20 hectares), the site selected for the park had been a farm where produce for those living at the House of Providence on Power Street was grown. Amusements at the park included a Shoot the Chutes, merry-go-round, scenic railway (roller coaster), Bump the Bumps, as well as a variety of food concessions, games of chance, side shows, plus a lacrosse field and bicycle track. The park's centrepiece was a 125-foot-high (38 metres) light tower at the base of which was a large restaurant. It was at the park in 1907 that pioneer aviator Charles Willard treated hundreds of Torontonians to their first look at a heavier-than-air flying machine. Seeing the value of the park as a source of income both from the rides and concessions as well as from fares paid to get to and from the park on their streetcars, the privately owned Toronto Railway Company purchased Scarboro' Beach and ran it until 1925 when the new municipally operated Toronto Transportation Commission refused to take it over. Soon after its closure, the rides and buildings were removed and "modestly priced houses, in the $5,400 to $7,500 range" were erected and offered for sale. As part of the land transfer a strip of land along the water's edge was retained by the city for future inclusion in what was described as the "Beaches waterfront park and athletic field," which wouldn't get built for nearly seven more years.

BALMY BEACH CANOE CLUB (163) has existed as a non-profit organization serving the residents of the Beach community since 1905, when members of the Beach Success hockey club formed a canoe club to help the members stay fit during the off season. They made a deal with a local boathouse owner and the Balmy Beach Canoe Club was born. The first club house was built on land formerly owned by Sir Adam Wilson, a larger-than-life lawyer, judge, and Toronto's first "elected" mayor (previous to Wilson's first term in 1859 the mayor was appointed by the members of city council). Unfortunately, that first club house was destroyed by fire in 1936, but soon a new facility took its place. History repeated itself in 1963 when the club house was again consumed by flames. The present structure opened two years later. Though, as the club's title suggests, in its earliest days canoeing was the main focus of the organization, today's membership enjoys football (in 1927 and 1930 the Balmy Beach team won the coveted Grey Cup, lawn bowling, rugby, hockey, squash, volleyball, basketball, and, wait

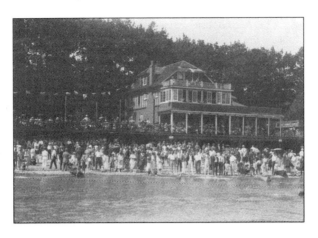

The old Balmy Beach Clubhouse, 1922.

for it, surfboarding! An interesting bit of Olympic sports trivia involves the Balmy Beach club, for when canoeing was introduced as an exhibition event in 1924 club member Roy Nurse won two gold and four bronze medals. One of the club's most popular members was the "Bard of Balmy Beach," Ted Reeve, a sports writer with the *Telegram* newspaper who created a trio of never-to-be-forgotten characters on the Toronto scene, Alice Snippersnapper, Moaner McGruffey, and Nutsy Fagan.

\* \* \* \* \*

## From the end of the Boardwalk proceed north on Silverbirch Avenue to Queen Street, then east to the R.C. Harris Filtration Plant

MUNRO PARK AVENUE is another example of how spelling mistakes occur even in the names of Toronto streets. Like Carlton (which should be "Carelton" as in Guy Carelton Wood), Sherbourne (for Sherborne, Dorsetshire, England), and Princess (was "Princes" for the nine sons of King George III), Munro should be "Monro" for George Monro, prominent businessman, successful politician (city alderman and mayor, MPP) and local landowner. A portion of his property, through which this street runs, was the site of a small, but highly successful amusement park from 1896 until 1907. When the park closed the land was subdivided, streets laid out, and houses built.

NEVILLE PARK BOULEVARD, which was laid out on the site of the park, recognizes Brent Neville, who married George Monro's daughter Frances Jane.

NURSEWOOD AVENUE honours the Nurse family, two members of which — Roy and Jerry — were champion paddlers who trained at the nearby Balmy Beach club.

R.C. HARRIS WATER TREATMENT PLANT (164): Because some thought the expenditure on this project was an incredible waste of the taxpayer's money, the R.C. Harris Water Filtration Plant was frequently called the "Palace of Purification." Today, many recognize the plant as an architectural masterpiece, one of the city's truly impressive treasures. Architect William Pomphrey would be proud to know the facility has been declared a National Historic Civil Engineering Site. The first supplier of water to the populace of Toronto was Albert Furniss, an entrepreneurial type who convinced the city fathers that he could do the job. His company, the Furniss Works, kept on supplying the city's water requirements for the next three decades until that responsibility was turned over to the city in 1873. To keep up with a growing city the filtration plant on Toronto Island (see 173) and the pumping station at the foot of John Street (see 48) were constantly being upgraded and miles and miles of water mains and numerous storage reservoirs added. The site on which the Harris plant sits was many years before a small summer pleasure ground known as Victoria Park, thus the name of the nearby street. The grounds opened in 1878 and were a popular attraction, accessible at first primarily by boat from the big city then, as the area developed, by horse-drawn, and later, electric streetcars. In 1906 the park ceased operating although for many years afterwards it was the site of one of the Toronto Board of Education's unique "forest schools" where the mental, moral, and physical development of the student could be greatly improved through prolonged contact with the natural environment. A similar school was also established in High Park. The idea of utilizing the Victoria Park site, which was actually outside the city in the Township of Scarborough (later a borough, then a city, and now part of Toronto) for a water filtration plant was first proposed by the newly appointed commissioner of the city's new Works Department. Rowland Caldwell Harris, who was born in the Toronto suburb of Lansing in 1875 and was first employed by the city as an office boy at the old, old City Hall on Front Street East at Jarvis. He worked his way through the ranks and in 1905, at the age of just 30, became Property Commissioner. Five years later he was appointed the Commissioner of Street Cleaning and when these two departments were combined in 1912 and a new Works Department was created Harris became its first commissioner. He died in 1945 at his residence at 10 Neville Park Boulevard, two blocks west of the plant that was to be named in his honour. Work on what at first was referred to simply as the Victoria Park waterworks plant commenced in 1932. Seven years later the new plant was in operation although the outbreak of war and the fear of sabotage (guards were posted and the windows covered to prevent tampering with the treated water) delayed the official opening until November 1, 1941 when Mayor Fred Conboy performed that task. Originally the plant processed a maximum of 100 million gallons (455 million litres) of raw water per day, obtained from Lake Ontario via an intake 50 feet (15 metres) below the surface and 8,695 feet (2,650 metres) from the shore line. Since then, with the growth of the city the volume has been increased several times (and a second intake added) so that today the plant is able to process 171.1 million gallons (650 million litres) per day. The R.C. Harris plant provides, on an annual basis, forty-five per cent of the total requirements of potable water for both the City of Toronto and much of the Regional Municipality of York located north of the city.

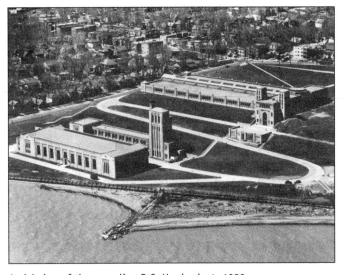

Aerial view of the sprawling R.C. Harris plant, 1952.


**End of Walk Two**

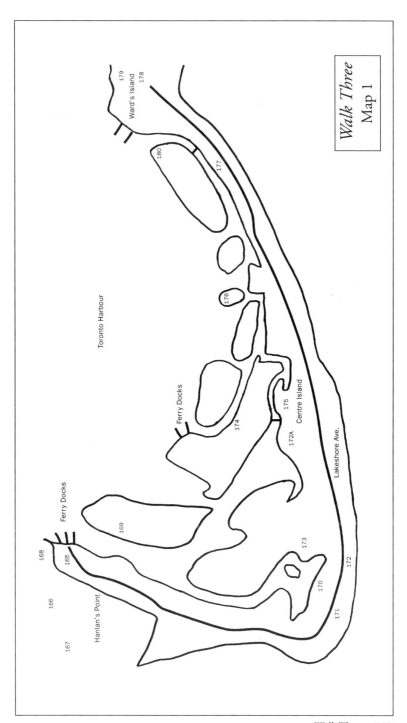

Walk Three
Map 1

Toronto Harbour

Ward's Island

179

178

180

177

176

174

175

172A

Centre Island

Lakeshore Ave.

Ferry Docks

Ferry Docks

168

165

169

166

167

Hanlan's Point

173

170

171

172

# Walk Three

## Toronto Bay and Toronto Island

Whether simply strolling along the water's edge or enjoying a leisurely crossing to or from the Island, visitors to the city's waterfront will see a multitude of pleasure and work craft on Toronto Bay each "doing its thing." Every one of these craft has its own interesting, and sometimes fascinating history.

### Yacht Club Passenger Vessels:

The oldest ship on Toronto Bay and believed to be the world's oldest active passenger vessel is the Royal Canadian Yacht Club's (RCYC) 65-foot (20-metre) ferry *HIAWATHA*. Built at a cost of $7,000 as a replacement for the RCYC's first launch, *Esperanza*, the "grand old lady of Toronto Bay" was launched in 1895 at the Bertram Engine Works yard at the foot of Bathurst Street, a site that, following extensive landfilling operations carried out earlier this century, is now buried several hundred feet inland. Named for the Algonquin deity and hero of Henry Wadsworth Longfellow's epic poem *Hiawatha* (written exactly forty years before little *Hiawatha* was launched), this vessel was originally steam powered, being converted to diesel in 1944. She underwent a major $150,000 facelift in 1982 that will ensure her presence on Toronto Bay for years to come.

*Hiawatha*'s running mate is *KWASIND*, a 71-foot (21.6-metre) launch built in 1912 at a cost of $20,000 by the Polson Iron Works Company at their yard at the foot of Princess Street on the old waterfront (another site that is now, as a result of landfilling, located well inland). Kwasind (meaning "very strong man") was the name of Hiawatha's friend in the famous poem. Both *Kwasind* and *Hiawatha* are used to shuttle club members to and from the RCYC's Island clubhouse dock and the mainland dock near the foot of Parliament Street.

Two other RCYC vessels are frequently seen on Toronto Bay: the tender *ELSIE D.*, which was a gift of a club member, and *ESPERANZA IV*, named in honour of the club's first launch, which was in service from 1881 until 1895. Today's *Esperanza* was built in less than a month in Owen Sound, Ontario, and first saw service as a Niagara Falls sightseeing vessel, *Little Maid of the Mist*. She was pressed into service after the *Maid of the Mist* burned at her Niagara River dock in 1956 and was sold following the arrival of two larger sightseeing boats.

Operating from York Street to their clubhouse on Mugg's Island, *DOC WILLINSKY* is the Island Yacht Club's launch. She was named for one of the founders of the IYC and prominent Toronto surgeon Dr. Bernard Willinsky. It was Dr. Willinsky's personal launch *Mona IV* that accompanied Marilyn Bell as she swam Lake Ontario in September, 1954 (see 109). The Island Yacht Club also operates two other small craft, *ISLAND PRINCE* and *IYC*. The Queen City Yacht Club operates *ALGONQUIN QUEEN* from city side to their club on Algonquin Island.

\* \* \* \* \*

Charter and sightseeing boats proliferate on Toronto Bay. Here are a few that have interesting histories:

## Charter and Tour Boats:

The newest charter boat is the *YANKEE LADY III*, which was built in the Ship Channel (see 139) and launched in 1997. With an overall length of 115 feet (35 metres) and drawing 27 feet (8.2 metres) of water the newest addition to the *Yankee Lady* fleet is the largest vessel built in Toronto since the ferry boat *Thomas Rennie* (see below) took to the water in 1951. She joins joining *YANKEE LADY I* (an American industrialist's personal yacht launched in 1965) and *YANKEE LADY II* (a former dive tender launched in 1981). Incidentally, the trio of *Yankee Ladies*, though with American sounding names are, in fact, owned by a Torontonian whose radio call sign was "Yankee Lady." The "sisters" are berthed at the foot of Jarvis Street from where they depart on charters and Sunday open cruises.

*CHALLENGE* is a 95-foot (30-metre) three-masted schooner built in 1980 in Port Stanley, Ontario, on the style of the original *Challenge,* the first clipper schooner on the Great Lakes which was built at Manitowac, Wisconsin in 1852.

*EMPIRE SANDY* was launched at Willington-Quay-on-Tyne, England in 1943 as one of a number of a "Empire" class ocean-going steam salvage tugs and was used primarily to haul disabled warships back to port. During the Second World War, the 143-foot (43.6-metre) vessel saw service in the Mediterranean Sea and Atlantic and Indian Oceans. In 1948, she was renamed *Ashford* and four years later began working for the Great Lakes Paper Company on Lake Superior and Lake of the Woods as the logging tug *Chris M.* In the early 1970s, just as she was headed for the scrap heap, the vessel was purchased and a major conversion programme initiated here in Toronto in 1975 that saw her lengthened 57 feet (17 metres) to 200 feet (61 metres) and renamed *Empire Sandy.* This impressive-looking craft, with 10,000 square feet (929 square metres) of sail (she is the largest sailing vessel in the country and she has an auxiliary 320 horsepower diesel engine, in case) provides a unique charter service on Toronto Bay. She is berthed at the Jarvis Street Slip.

*PATHFINDER* and *PLAYFAIR* are operated by Toronto Brigantine, a non-profit youth training organization incorporated in 1964. Both vessels are 60 feet (18 metres) in length, have steel hulls, and are two-masted with square-rigged sails on the foremast. *Pathfinder* was launched in 1964, *Playfair* in 1974.

*SHIPSANDS* is a fifty-one-passenger, diesel-powered tour boat operated by Toronto Tours from a berth at the foot of York Street. Built in Meaford, Ontario, in 1972, the vessel's name comes from the fact that in her previous life as a tour boat operating out of Moosonee in Northern Ontario, *Shipsands* would frequently take tourists past the Ship Sands Island bird sanctuary in James Bay. This island was so named because ships running out of Moosonee, empty after having dropped off their cargo, would remove sand from the island for ballast. *Shipsands* also served as a "school bus" at certain times of the year, taking children from Moose Factory Island to their school on the mainland. The craft was acquired by Toronto Tours in 1984 and transported to Toronto where she was lengthened from 40 feet (12 metres) to 46 feet (14 metres) the following year.

Toronto Tours also operates the *KIM SIMPSON,* which was built in Holland in 1956 and was seen on the canals of Amsterdam for several years prior to being shipped to her new home here on Toronto Bay.

The company also has the *HARRY G. KIMBER*, a 45-foot (14-metre) launch powered by twin 440 cubic inch (7,210 cubic centimetre) gas engines built in 1965 here in Toronto by the Taylor boat works at their yard near the foot of Bathurst Street. The craft was named for a former Toronto Harbour Commissioner.

Mariposa Cruise Lines operates a number of cruise boats on the bay. They are *MATTHEW FLINDERS, EMPRESS OF CANADA, SHOWBOAT, NORTHERN SPIRIT, TORONTONIAN, MARIPOSA BELLE,* and *ORIOLE.* The latter craft, 75 feet (23 metres) in length, was built in 1987 in Port Dover, Ontario, on the style of a "Victorian-era Canadian riverboat." All are berthed at Harbourfront Centre.

## Toronto Island Ferries:

The Toronto Parks Department has a monopoly on passenger ferry service to and from Toronto Island (as did the TTC who ran the service until 1962 using streetcar tickets as fares). Parks operates a fleet of five double-end vessels from docks at the foot of Bay Street (see 26), directly south of the Harbour Castle Hotel. Four of the ferries operate to three Toronto Island destinations — Ward's Island, Centre Island, and Hanlan's Point — throughout most of the year with more frequent departures during the warmer months. Be aware that in the winter only the Ward's Island boat operates, on a much-reduced schedule.

The flagship of the fleet is the restored 150-foot (46-metre) steam-powered, side-paddle *TRILLIUM*, launched at the Polson Iron Works yard at the foot of Princess Street on June 18, 1910. Built at a cost of $75,000 and with an initial passenger capacity of 1,350 (now reduced to 900 for safety), *Trillium* was retired in 1956, but was returned to service, complete with her original steam engine powering twin side-paddles, in 1976 following a $1-million municipally funded restoration program. *Trillium* operates primarily in charter service, but does assist the three other Island ferries during peak periods in the summer.

The second oldest is *WILLIAM INGLIS*, named for a prominent Toronto businessman and the president of the John Inglis Company that built the vessel in 1935. Originally the vessel was to be named *Shamrock* to continue a forty-five-year tradition of naming Island ferries after flowers (*Mayflower* and *Primrose* in 1890, *Blue Bell* in 1906, and *Trillium* in 1910). The 99-foot (30-metre) diesel-powered vessel was actually put into service in 1936 as the *William Inglis* in tribute to Inglis who died in November of 1935, just months before the craft his company built was to enter regular Island ferry service.

In 1939, *SAM McBRIDE*, another diesel-powered, though slightly longer ferry at 129 feet (39.3 metres), entered service allowing the retirement and scrapping of the two forty-nine-year-old ferries *Mayflower* and *Primrose*. The *Sam McBride* was named for a popular Toronto mayor (and long-time Island resident) who first served as the chief magistrate in 1928–1929 and was re-elected to the position again in 1936. Sam McBride died while still in office and city council honoured his memory by naming the new vessel after him.

In 1951, a sister ship to the *Sam McBride* (identical in all respects), was added to the fleet. This one was christened *THOMAS RENNIE*, after a prominent Toronto businessman and long-time Harbour Commissioner.

The last three vessels were all built in Toronto by the John Inglis Company. The fifth and smallest vessel was built in Owen Sound in 1963 and is named *ONGIARA*, a form of either "Onghiara" or "Onguiaahra," an Amerindian words that translates as either "thundering waters" or "the straits," respectively. It's believed that either word could also be the source of the word Niagara. In the summer *Ongiara* is used primarily as a freight boat. In the winter months it's in service when traffic is at its lightest. *Ongiara* is also able to navigate the crossing to Ward's if and when the Bay becomes ice-covered. Call 392-8193 for ferry schedule details and 392-8188 for charter information.

## Toronto City Centre Airport Ferries:

A visit to the Toronto City Centre Airport at Hanlan's Point, whether to catch a plane or just for a visit, also requires the use of a ferry. In this case it's the 64-foot (19.5-metre), one-hundred-passenger (and up to six cars) double-end ferry *MAPLE CITY*, which departs regularly from her dock just west of the foot of Bathurst Street. Built in Port Dalhousie, Ontario, in 1951, she originally operated between Prescott, Ontario, and Ogdensburg, New York. In 1965 she arrived in Toronto and began a new career ferrying passengers on a two-minute trip between the mainland dock just west of the foot of Bathurst Street and the Island Airport dock 400 feet (122-metres) across the Western Gap. This hardy little craft is on duty sixteen hours a day, seven days a week and usually operates on a fifteen-minute schedule. When *Maple City* commenced her Island Airport run in 1965 she replaced a small "no name" cable ferry that had initiated service shortly after the airport opened in 1937. When necessary, *Windmill Point*, out of Amherstburg, Ontario, replaces *Maple City* on one of the world's shortest ferry routes.

\* \* \* \* \*

## Work Boats:

It's not all fun and games on Toronto Bay. A few of the busiest and most frequently seen work boats are described below.

The Toronto Harbour Commission (THC) tug *WILLIAM REST* was launched at Erieau, Ontario in 1961 and is named for a long-time Commission employee. Bill Rest joined the THC in 1915 and died in 1961 shortly after being appointed to the position of Director of Planning. The name of the work boat *FRED SCANDRETT* recalls the THC's general manager from 1946 to 1951. An interesting yet unsung member of the THC's fleet is *Derrick No. 50*, built by the American Corps of Engineers in the early 1950s. Here in Toronto the craft was used up until the mid-1970s to off-load container cargo at Marine Terminals 51 & 52 from the water side of the dock, thus saving both time and labour. The THC also operates *Kenneth A,* a 40-foot (12-metre) work boat built in the early 1960s.

One of the busiest tugs on the Bay is the Toronto Works Department's 42-foot (13-metre), 180 HP diesel-powered *NED HANLAN II* which was launched at Erieau, Ontario in 1966. This vessel is the successor to the first tug of that name which in turn was named in honour of Toronto-born Ned Hanlan (1855-1908) one of the world's foremost scullers. The original *Ned Hanlan* is moored at The Pier at the west end of Harbourfront Centre.

Occasionally seen on the bay are the work tugs *COLLINETTE* and *DUCHESS V.* The former, 65 feet (20 metres) in length and powered by a 600 HP diesel engine, was built for the Royal Canadian Navy in 1944 in Owen Sound, Ontario, and originally named *Lac Ottawa.* Years later she crossed the Atlantic Ocean under her own power and worked as a docking tug in various English ports. Returning to Canada in the mid-1950s, this time as deck cargo, the tug was purchased by Waterman's Services and renamed *Collinette* after two members of the owner's family, Colin and Janette. *Duchess V*, 55 feet (17 metres) in length with a 700 HP diesel engine, was launched at Owen Sound in 1955 and worked her first few years on Lake Superior and Lake of the Woods as the logging tug *Anglo Duchess.* Both *Colinette* and *Duchess V* are operated by Waterman's Services, a company that has been in the business of looking after the needs of visiting ships for more than forty years.

\* \* \* \* \*

# Around Toronto Island:

A tour of Toronto's fascinating waterfront wouldn't be complete with a trip to Toronto Island, a short fifteen-minute ferry boat trip across Toronto Bay. Originally Toronto Island was a long, narrow peninsula along with a few "whisps" of land, all of which were created over eons of time as a result of the continual erosion of the Bluffs at Scarborough to the east of the city. A strong and persistent Lake Ontario current carried the eroded material from the base of the Bluffs in a westerly direction. When the outflow from the Humber River was encountered the lake current slowed and the silt settled out of suspension forming a hook-like peninsula that was joined to the mainland at the east end by a narrow isthmus. On April 13, 1858, a violent storm caused the Don River to become a raging torrent that, combined with mountainous waves on the lake, washed through this isthmus, seperating the peninsula from the mainland. Toronto Island was born. Today, as a result of landfilling operations carried out by the Toronto Harbour Commission since its inception in the early teens, the Island has been increased in size to more than 820 acres (328 hectares) of land and lagoons. To be absolutely accurate the use of the singular noun "Island" is incorrect since the modern-day Toronto Island actually consists of eighteen islets of various sizes separated by a series of lagoons.

The first people to visit what is now referred to as Toronto Island were the Mississauga Indians who, suffering from war wounds or sickness, recognized the recuperative powers afforded by the peninsula and took refuge under the shady trees or bathed in the peninsula's cool lagoons. Their early presence was recorded on maps of the time that gave the name Hiawatha to the peninsula. Following European settlement of the Town of York across the bay in the late 1700s, visitors to the peninsula frequently rode there on horseback. One of those visitors, Elizabeth Simcoe, wife of the city's founder, wrote in her diary about riding to what she called "her favourite sands." In the depths of winter, when the clear waters of the Bay froze solid, people could simply walk to the peninsula.

As early as 1833 an enterprising Michael O'Connor began a ferry boat service with his first craft, called the *John of the Peninsula*, a two-horsepower craft powered by (what else?) two horses walking on a circular-shaped treadmill. The rotating motion of this treadmill was transferred by gears and shafts to sidepaddles on either side of the craft. These paddles propelled the little craft from the town wharf near the foot of Church Street to O'Connor's Hotel on the peninsula and back. With the breaching of the narrow isthmus connecting the peninsula with the mainland in 1858, access to the newly created island was almost exclusively by ferry boat. Before long dozens of ferry boats arrived on the bay, where business was both brisk and lucrative. Now, more than a century later, ferry boats (albeit of the more modern variety) continue the tradition of providing "less-than-rapid" transit to the Island. Let's board one and, because we have to start somewhere, journey to the most westerly part of the Island, Hanlan's Point. Be sure to check on the times boats return to the mainland. Otherwise you may be stuck under the stars overnight — not bad in the summer, but awfully cold in the winter.

## Hanlan's Point (* indicates Hanlan's Point sites):

In days gone by, Hanlan's was the busiest, and noisiest, place on the Island. One of the popular myth's in Toronto's history is that this part of the Island was named for Toronto's famous sculler Edward "Ned" Hanlan. In fact, this part of Toronto Island was named for his father John, an Irish immigrant who settled first at Owen Sound on Georgian Bay. John eventually moved to Toronto, settling at the east end of the peninsula where he built a small clapboard shack for his wife Ann and himself. A severe storm struck the Island sometime in 1865 and washed the Hanlan home, with the family huddled inside (a family that now included two sons, John Jr. and Edward), into Toronto Bay. After an exciting voyage the family and their "houseboat" washed ashore at the west end of the Island. John proceeded to build a new family home on land that would be officially deeded to him the next year. As a result, this part of the Island became known as Hanlan's Point. A few years later, Hanlan built a small hotel to accommodate the increasing number of visitors venturing over to the Island from the mainland. His son Ned, who was born at the old General Hospital at the northwest corner of King Street West at John Street in 1855, would become a highly talented sculler primarily because he lived on the Island. Back then the first person to bring fish they'd caught in the waters off Toronto Island over to the St. Lawrence Market (and an eager and waiting public) would be the first to sell his fish. Therefore, the better the salesman's sculling talents, the better the financial return. And Ned was *the* best. He won numerous sculling competitions, including the World's Championship in 1880. It that same year Ned invested some of his victory earnings in a new and larger hotel at Hanlan's Point. Before long an amusement park complete with rides and food stands began to develop nearby.

* HANLAN'S POINT AMUSEMENT PARK (site of, 165): The park became a favourite for Torontonians and grew rapidly. In addition to the rides, games, and food concessions, a new stadium opened in the park in 1897. Unfortunately, the hometown Maple Leaf baseball team lost their opening encounter with the team from Rochester 11–0. A sad event occurred on the afternoon of August 10, 1909, when a small fire broke out in the park's Gem Theatre. The building was tinder dry and the flames quickly

roared out of control. By the time the blaze was extinguished several hours later the hotel, many of the park's buildings and rides, as well as the old stadium all lay in ruins. The saddest news was that the young theatre cashier had succumbed to her burns. A new stadium, this time made of concrete, was quickly erected on the site of the old and it was here that on Saturday, September 5, 1914, a young rookie pitcher playing for the Providence Grays, George Herman "Babe" Ruth, hit his first professional home run over the right field bleachers into Toronto Bay. The event is commemorated by a historic plaque affixed to a rock not far from the Hanlan's Point ferry dock. In 1926, the ball team moved to the new stadium at the foot of Bathurst Street over on the mainland (see 65). The amusement park skidded downhill with the once-popular stadium finally coming to a rather sad end with its unceremonious demolition in 1937. A few of the rides and a large roller rink managed to survive into the 1950s, but now they too are gone.

Retired Island ferry *Trillium* crosses the bay in December, 1973 as restoration work begins.

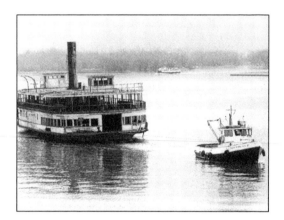

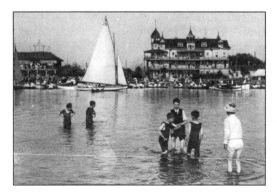

The pleasures of Hanlan's Point, Toronto's "Coney Island," circa 1900.

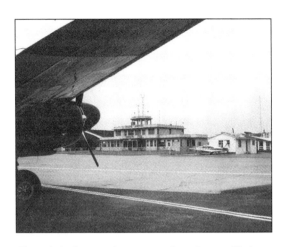

The original control tower at Port George VI (now Toronto City Centre) Airport has been retained.

* WEST END BATHS (site of, 166): This early "water park" was developed by Peter McIntyre in 1884 and consisted of men's and women's change rooms, a 500-foot (152-metre) stretch of Lake Ontario waterfront and a water slide (known then as a "shoot"). The baths, which eventually became known as Turner's Baths, were extremely popular until abandoned in favour of a new public bathing beach that opened nearby in the mid-1930s.

* TORONTO CITY CENTRE AIRPORT (167): At the same time the Hanlan's Point Amusement Park was going into decline, plans were being finalized by the Toronto Harbour Commission to build a new airport at Hanlan's Point. The new facility opened in 1939 and was officially designated as the Port George VI Airport, recognizing the fact that it opened the same year that King George VI and Queen Elizabeth paid their first visit to the city. The idea of building an airport at the Island (along with an emergency field near the Village of Malton northwest of the city should fog or some other occurrence prohibit the use of the Island facility) first surfaced in the early 1930s. However, work on Toronto's new Island Airport didn't start until 1937 when Toronto Harbour Commission crews began removing cottages (some of which were taken over the ice that winter to what is now called Algonquin Island far to the east), levelling the amusement park and filling in lagoons on which landing and taxiing strips were laid out and a control tower built. Included in the original drawings was a tunnel from the foot of Bathurst Street to a parking lot adjacent to the new airport. Needless to say, that tunnel was not to be.

While work was going full steam ahead at the Island site, the Harbour Commission was also busy constructing the alternate airport at Malton. Today, this airport, now greatly enlarged and modernized, is known as Lester B. Pearson International Airport, even though most long-time Torontonians still refer to it simply as Malton Airport. This facility, which many said was too far from the city to work, was first used in the summer of 1938 with the arrival of an American Airlines DC-3 from Buffalo, New York, bringing officials to that year's Canadian National Exhibition. Toronto Island Airport, with an administration and control tower building built to the same specifications as the one out at Malton, welcomed its first official arrival in February of 1939. Later that year, the airport's first commercial flight landed bringing band leader Tommy Dorsey and his band to town for a performance at the Ex. Over the next eleven months, the Island Airport had slightly more than seven thousand take-offs and landings.

During the early part of the Second World War, the Island Airport became a training base for the members of the Royal Norwegian Air Force, who were billeted across the gap at Little Norway (see 63). In 1982, a STOL (short take-off and landing) commuter service between Toronto Island Airport and the airports at Ottawa and Montreal, was introduced using four-engine DASH 7s and later twin-engine DASH 8 commuter aircraft both types designed and built by Toronto's de Havilland Aircraft Company. Today, air operations are handled in a modern control tower that was put into service in 1987. To emphasize the airport's proximity to the downtown core, the airport has been known as Toronto City Centre Airport since 1994. There are now approximately 120,000 take-offs and landings annually.

* The CURTIS FLYING SCHOOL (site of, 168) was situated at the west end of the bay and adjacent to the site of the future Island Airport. It was Canada's first flying school and went into operation on May 10, 1915, with a fleet of three Curtis Type F flying-boat biplanes. In its first year the school turned out sixty-seven pilots, many of whom would make the supreme sacrifice during the Great War.

* BLOCKHOUSE BAY was so named for the nearby small wooden blockhouse erected nearby by Governor Simcoe to help protect the entrance into Toronto Harbour. Soon after Simcoe had established his provisional capital at York in 1793, he instructed that this blockhouse, complete with cannons and storehouse, be erected on the peninsula at a place he called Gibraltar Point, so-named because Simcoe felt it could be "fortified so as to be impregnable." The gun at this blockhouse, in combination with those at the newly constructed Fort York across the way, would guard his town from any invaders, or so Simcoe believed. How wrong he was. (see 117).

*  MUGG'S ISLAND, just across Blockhouse Bay from Hanlan's Point, was originally known as Mugg's Landing. Its unusual name first appeared in the 1880s when four young bachelors, who had decided to make the yet-unnamed small island the site of their personal summer "resort," complete with a couple of pitched tents, found a sign floating face up on the waters of Toronto Bay. It was advertising a play on the stage of the Royal Opera House on King Street West. The title of the play ... *Mugg's Landing*.

*  The ISLAND YACHT CLUB (IYC)(169) is on Mugg's Island and fronts on Blockhouse Bay. The club, which was established on this site in 1952 now has a membership of approximately four hundred members and is home port to almost two hundred yachts.

*  Continuing on our journey the ancient GIBRALTAR POINT LIGHTHOUSE soon comes into view (170). Completed in 1808, the 70-foot-high (21 metres) structure of Queenston, Ontario limestone is the oldest lighthouse on the Great Lakes. In 1832, the height of the lighthouse was increased by an additional 12 feet (3.7 metres) to its present 82 feet (25 metres). Now located well inland, the lighthouse was actually built right on the shore of Lake Ontario. Subsequent landfilling has "pushed" the structure further and further inland, or so it appears. Obviously, the structure hasn't moved an inch, while the man-made shoreline has. For more than fifteen decades the lighthouse guided shipping around the treacherous sandbars south of what at first was a peninsula and is now an island thanks to a vicious storm that breached the isthmus in April of 1858, creating a narrow gap between the new Toronto Island and the mainland. Remarkably, the old lighthouse remained in service until as recently as 1959. Legend has it that the ghost of the first lighthouse keeper, J.P. Radenmuller, who was murdered by a couple of troops from Fort York after he refused to share the contents of his liquor locker with them, still frequents the lighthouse. Ghosts. Bah! Incidentally, the term Gibraltar Point was penned by Governor Simcoe as it reminded him, in terms of its defensibility, of Gibraltar at the entrance to the Mediterranean Sea.

*  LAKESIDE HOME FOR CHILDREN (site of, 171), located just to the southwest of the lighthouse, came into being in 1883 thanks to the persistence of Elizabeth McMaster, one of the founders of Toronto's now world-famous Hospital for Sick Children. Money to build this pleasant summer retreat on the Island for the tiny patients of the children's hospital came from John Ross Robertson, founder of the *Evening Telegram* newspaper and one of the city's greatest benefactors. He had a particular interest in the welfare of children, having lost his infant daughter in 1881 to the ravages of scarlet fever. The Lakeside Home was such a success that

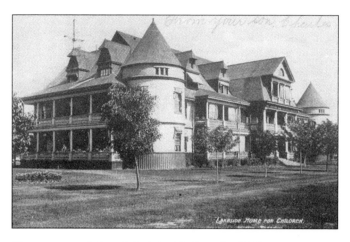

Vintage postcard view of the Lakeside Home for Children, 1907.

Robertson agreed to underwrite a major $40,000 expansion and renovation program that was completed in 1891. This enlarged structure was severely damaged by fire in April, 1915, and again Robertson came forward to pay for needed repairs. Every summer the children were transported to their summer home on the Island by the little Island ferryboat *Luella*. This tradition ended in 1928 when the Hospital for Sick Children's country facility at Thistletown, 13 miles (21 kilometres) northwest of Toronto, opened. The deserted Island buildings saw brief use in the early part of the Second World War as quarters for some Royal Norwegian Air Force flyers while Little Norway (see 63) on the mainland was being built. Then, following the war, the Lakeside Home was pressed into use as a wartime housing facility called Chetwood Terrace. The historic old structure was torn down in the mid-1950s.

\* \* \* \* \*

\* The TORONTO ISLAND PUBLIC/NATURAL SCIENCE SCHOOL (172) was originally established as a simple one-room schoolhouse in 1888 where seventeen children who lived year-round on the Island could learn the three "Rs". The first few years saw the little school closed for lack of funds on several occasions, but by 1896 the school had finally become a part of the Toronto Board of Education's annual budget. Sadly, the tiny school was destroyed by fire in 1905. However, a new one-room facility was soon in place which, in 1923, was doubled in size. A third room was added in 1932 with another room added some sixteen years later.

Following the end of the Second World War, a severe housing shortage hit Toronto that resulted in a large migration of citizens across Toronto Bay where they were able to take up residence in the numerous houses scattered across the Island. This resulted in increased enrollment at the Island School, which peaked at 587 students in 1954. On January 1, 1956, the Municipality of Metropolitan Toronto assumed responsibility for Toronto Island and quickly began terminating leases held on all Centre Island and Hanlan's Point properties. As people began vacating their Island homes, which were then bulldozed into oblivion, enrollment at the Island school plummeted. In 1960, the school was converted into a Natural Science School where sixty-eight Grade 5 and 6 students from the mainland could come for a week of learning in the great "out-of-doors."

Today, some of the schoolrooms continue to be devoted to the teaching of junior kindergarten through to Grade 6 for the remaining Island and a few mainland students. There is also a day nursery for fifteen children ages 2–5 as well as a parenting centre for pre-school children and their caregivers. To meet the needs of a growing school population, both here on the Island as well as an increasing demand from the mainland, a new $7.5 million Island Public and Natural Science School is presently (1998) under construction nearby. Following a three-year selection process the Toronto architectural firm of Robbie Sane was selected. It is anticipated that the new school, described as "a rustic wood building consisting of discrete but connected elements sitting low in the landscape" will open in the winter of 1998, at which time the old school will be demolished. Incorporated into the new school design will be such environmentally friendly features as a grey water reclamation and recycling system, composting of kitchen wastes and an exterior wetlands demonstration area.

* TORONTO ISLAND FILTRATION PLANT (173): East of the lighthouse is the Toronto Island Filtration Plant, the fourth such plant on this site. The first opened in 1874 and consisted of a rather simple infiltration basin 2,700 feet (823 metres) in length, 470 feet (143 metres) wide and 14 feet (4.3 metres) deep. This operation was able to supply Toronto's 67,995 citizens with 4.5 million gallons (20.5 million litres) of filtered water per day. The water was transferred to the mainland through a wooden pipe 4 feet (1.2 metres) in diameter which was laid across the Island from the filtration plant and connected to a 3-foot (1-metre) cast iron pipe under Toronto Bay. In 1909, work started on a 39.6-million-gallon (180-million-litre) slow sand filtration plant that opened in late 1911 and remained in service until 1968 and on standby until 1975. Water for this and subsequent plants was drawn from Lake Ontario. A third plant went on stream in December, 1917, and was able to supply a population that had risen to 473,829 with an additional 60 million gallons (273 million litres) of

water purified by a mechanical drifting sand filter process. This plant was in operation until 1977 and decommissioned in 1981. Portions of the 1911 and 1917 plants are still visible. The present plant, and fourth on the site, is of the modern, high rate, direct filtration variety and was placed in service in 1977. When in service it is able to operate at a maximum capacity of 60 million gallons (273 million litres) per day. Filtered water flows to the John Street Pumping Station through a huge 8-foot (2.4-metre) horseshoe-shaped tunnel carved through the bedrock beneath Toronto Bay. While the first three Island filtration plants operated year-round, new filtration plants constructed along the waterfront and the upgrading of the huge R.C. Harris Filtration Plant (see 164) on Queen Street East have resulted in the present Island facility operating only during peak demand periods from May 1 to October 1 each year.

## Centre Island (* indicates Centre Island sites):

Leaving Hanlan's Point and proceeding east along the shore of Lake Ontario, the Island visitor eventually arrives at that part of Toronto Island that gets its name from being, wait for it, in the approximate centre of one long island that stretches from Hanlan's Point on the west to Ward's Island on the east. Today's Centre Island evolved from what was originally a pleasure garden called Island Park that had been established by city council in 1880. Island Park sat on land given to the citizens by the Crown soon after Canada came into being in 1867. Soon a number of civic improvements were underway including walkways, docking facilities, and the planting of flowers and shrubs. Then, in the latter years of the last century, something extraordinary began to happen. What had been classified as a park was soon ringed with houses, many of which were of the beautifully ornate variety, two- and three-storey structures erected by some of the elite city citizens across the bay. For them Toronto Island had become their "Rosedale across the bay." Other more ordinary looking residences began to appear and before long a full-fledged community, complete with several hotels, stores, a fire hall, police station, theatre, and dance hall, and, stretching from Hanlan's Point to the western edge of Ward's Island, had taken hold. The population of the Island community reached more than ten thousand thanks to the severe housing shortage over on the mainland that followed the end of the Second World War. That living, breathing community flourished until the new Metropolitan government, created in 1953, was ordered to restore Toronto Island to its original status of public park. In 1956 the bulldozers arrived and by the spring of 1959, notwithstanding numerous demonstrations by concerned Islanders and others, the once-thriving Centre Island community was no more.

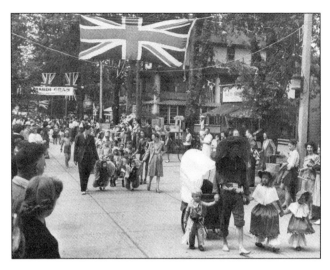

Children's Mardi Gras street parade on Manitou Road, Centre Island, 1953.

By 1961, the spanking clean AVENUE OF THE ISLANDS had replaced Manitou Road, Centre Island's once-bustling main street. A walk along the lakefront will reveal to the explorer a few remaining concrete walkways in front of Centre Island's phantom houses. Ferries to the mainland depart from the Centre Island dock, just to the north. Northwest of the dock is the Toronto Island Marina, a public boating facility with approximately five hundred mooring slips that opened in Canada's centennial year, 1967.

* CENTREVILLE (174), a lovely children's amusement park in a turn-of-the-century village setting, also opened in Canada's centennial year, 1967, and over the years has evolved into one of the main features of Centre Island. The showpiece of Centreville is a 1898 merry-go-round that replaced a home-grown version that was unceremoniously thrown out when "old" things weren't regarded as "in" things. There's also a flume ride and a picturesque Skyride.

* One of the special attractions of Centreville is its marvellous 3-acre (1.2-hectare) FAR ENOUGH FARM, a kind of country farm in the city. It received its unique name when the Metro Parks Commissioner of the day, the late Tommy Thompson, while surveying the future farm site, heard a mother address her young charges with the statement, "Let's go home, we've walked far enough."

*   Nearby, over a quaint arched bridge, is OLYMPIC ISLAND, once known as Toothpick Island before major reclamation by the city's Parks Department in the early years of this century expanded that toothpick into an extremely popular athletic ground. It is the perfect vantage point for a stunning view of the city's skyline.

*   Continuing our tour of the Island, we again head east and soon arrive in front of a charming little church. ST. ANDREW'S-BY-THE-LAKE (175) was built in 1884 as an outreach parish by the congregation of the city's first house of worship, St. James' Anglican Church at the northeast corner of King and Church streets in downtown Toronto. St. Andrew's-by-the-Lake originally stood to the west of the present Avenue of the Islands where it served the religious needs of the vibrant Island community. Then in 1959, even as the demolition of the Centre Island homes was well underway, the historic little church was carefully moved to its present location. And praised be ... it's still "in business." Now non-denominational, it is the site of numerous weddings and a variety of community events.

*   The ROYAL CANADIAN YACHT CLUB (176) sits on two islands (two of the nearly two dozen that make up what's referred to in the singular as Toronto Island) just north of the church. This private club was established in 1852 as the Toronto Boat Club with "fees of $2 per annum." Five months later, the name was changed to the Toronto Yacht Club. The prefix "Royal" and the alteration from "Toronto" to "Canadian" were approved in a letter sent to the club from Queen Victoria in 1854 and while the prefix "Royal" had been requested, no one knows how the word "Canadian" got into the title. The alteration wasn't questioned, however. In fact, questioning Queen Victoria at all was out of the question. From its inception, the RCYC has always met somewhere on Toronto's waterfront. First, it was in a one-storey wooden structure erected on top of a scow floating at the foot of Rees Street. One day the scow sank, but fortunately the club members had sensed something was amiss and had already moved to a new meeting place. This time it was on board the ancient steamer *Provincial*, which the club had recently purchased in Buffalo, New York, and towed to the Toronto waterfront. Following several sinkings and a few unauthorized sailings by this steamer-cum-clubhouse during stormy weather, a new, more permanent home was found in 1869 in a building straddling the end of the Simcoe Street wharf. With the arrival of the railways and resulting alterations to the layout of the waterfront, the RCYC was again forced to find a new site for its clubhouse. This time a location across the Island was suggested and after considerable debate amongst the members, both for and against the proposed move to "the wilds of Toronto Island," a site consisting mostly of marsh lands was chosen and in 1880 a

twenty-one-year, fifty-dollar annual lease was signed. Before another year had passed additional land had been reclaimed from the marsh and a new Island clubhouse was erected. It was officially opened by that year's commodore of the club (and a future Toronto mayor), Arthur Boswell. Unfortunately, this new clubhouse lasted only twenty-three years, for on the evening of August 15, 1904, just four short months after fire had wiped out most of downtown Toronto, the fire fiend returned. In less than thirty minutes, a small blaze in the rafters of the club's ornate wooden structure mushroomed into a roaring conflagration that quickly destroyed the structure. Nothing daunted, within two years another new and substantially larger building was ready for business on the site of the club's first Island clubhouse. But this one only lasted a dozen years, for it too was consumed by fire. The cornerstone of the third, and present clubhouse was laid by the Prince of Wales during his visit to Toronto in the summer of 1919. This structure, designed by the well-known Toronto architectural firm of Sproatt and Rolph, was built at a cost of $115,911 and was officially opened by Commodore George Gooderham on June 22, 1922. George Gooderham was a direct descendant of the founder of Gooderham and Worts distillery empire (see 1) and the builder of the King Edward Hotel on King Street East in 1903. Incidentally, some of the cannons on the front lawn of the RCYC, which seem to point menacingly towards the city, were used in the Crimean War. Nearby is the memorial capstan, unveiled in the fall of 1926 by the governor general and dedicated to the memory of many club members who made the supreme sacrifice during the First World War. The inscription reads "They shall be remembered as long as the sun shines on the lawn of the Royal Canadian Yacht Club."

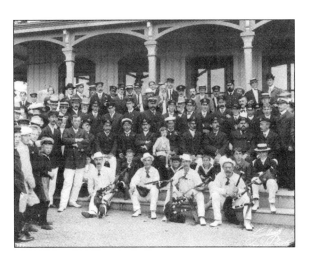

Members of the Royal Canadian Yacht Club pose for the photographer in front of the original Toronto Island clubhouse, circa 1900.

* TORONTO FIRE DEPARTMENT ISLAND FIRE HALL (177):
This fire hall, the creation of Toronto architect Paul Jurecka, opened in
1996 to serve not only the residents of Ward's and Algonquin Island, but
the station's firefighters are also capable of responding quickly to any
mishaps that might occur at the Toronto City Centre Airport. Interesting
features of the station's clock are the minute and hour hands represented by
a lightning bolt and a trident, respectively. These items symbolize the two
formidable opponents of fire and water. The four bronze faces at the 3, 6, 9,
and 12 positions represent man amused, man sleeping, man hiding, and
man alarmed. The other hour positions are defined by other objects — a
bird, a candle, a star, a house, a cloud, etc. What combination of objects will
the hands be singling out at the moment the station's alarm cries out? This
work is by Toronto artist Gord Peteran. A brochure describing the clock face
is available at the station.

## Ward's Island ( * indicates Ward's Island sites):

The third, and most easterly component of Toronto Island is Ward's.
It's named for David Ward who was born in Yarmouth, England, in 1817
and emigrated to Toronto in the 1830s taking up residence in a small shack
that the young man built on the Island when it was still a peninsula. Ward
was the foreman on the first horseboat that ran from the mainland to the
first hotel on the Island, and supplemented his income by fishing. David
Ward died at his Island residence in 1881.

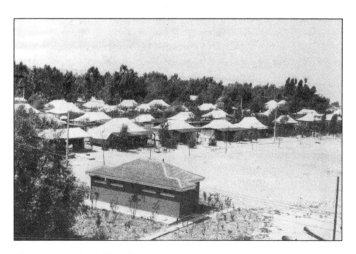

"Tent City," Ward's Island, 1923.

Ward's Island was the earliest part of Toronto Island to be developed with Michael O'Connor building his RETREAT ON THE PENINSULA hotel in 1833 (approx. site of 178). For a short period of time, this hotel was the summer home of Upper and Lower Canada's governor general, Lord Sydenham, who used it as his retreat from the dreaded cholera that had overwhelmed the community across the bay several times in the 1830s and 1840s. Over the next few years, the hotel was owned by a succession of hoteliers until, with a sign reading "Quinn's Hotel" over the door, it was swept away during the great storm of 1858 — the same storm that washed away the narrow isthmus connecting the peninsula with the mainland, thereby creating Toronto Island.

   \* WARD'S HOTEL (site of, 179) was another popular hostelry and was built by David's son William. Opened in 1883, the three-storey building had a look-out tower, an absolute essential if one was to sell liquor over the counter illegally. Over the years, the hotel was unsympathetically altered several times and then was used as a grocery store and snack bar before being demolished in 1966. Near the hotel were the Wiman Baths, erected in 1882 as a gift to the city from a former Toronto alderman, one Erasmus Wiman. Wiman had emigrated to the States several years earlier where he had done extremely well financially. In 1883, the baths (we'd call it a swimming pool today) were enlarged and in 1885 a quaint shelter added and the whole area landscaped. The entire attraction was flattened in the mid-1950s to make way for more park space. In 1899, the city began offering lots at Ward's at ten dollars a season. Soon a smattering of tents began unfolding each summer, a smattering that eventually grew into much larger numbers as citizens began to realize that the Island was a good place to "get away from it all." In 1913, city officials began re-arranging the tents into streets. Soon the tents were abandoned and wooden structures of all shapes and sizes took their place. Then in the mid-1930s, the city began offering annual leases and a decade later began encouraging the tenants to make improvements to alleviate the housing shortage that followed the end of the Second World War. With the transfer of the Island to Metro jurisdiction in 1956 and the authorization to develop the entire Island (except for the various yacht club properties and the airport) into parklands, plans to clear the entire Island of all houses were formulated. Work progressed at Centre and Hanlan's, but the Ward's and Algonquin Islanders didn't give in so quickly. Following years of often heated wrangling between the "let them stay, there's plenty of parkland" side, made up of City of Toronto officials and Toronto Island residents, and the "get them off the Island, we need more parkland" side, comprised of representatives of the Metropolitan Toronto government, the future of the communities on Ward's and Algonquin was settled in 1991 when the provincial government passed Bill 61 permitting the Islanders to lease their homes for a period of ninety-nine years. After another four years of working out the wording on the documents plus establishing a land trust to administer the whole matter, the first of the 250 or so leases was finally signed on April 11, 1995.

  * ALGONQUIN ISLAND, though not signed as a destination at the mainland ferry docks, is a co-community with that at Ward's. Algonquin Island is a relative newcomer to the Toronto Island scene, having grown out of a much smaller piece of property originally called Sunfish Island. The Algonquin community came into being at about the same time the new Toronto Island Airport at Hanlan's Point was in its early construction phase. To preserve some of the local cottages it was decided to move some of them to a new location closer to Ward's. Little Sunfish Island was selected as the new location and with extensive landfilling the small island was enlarged sufficiently to take the thirty or so houses that were to be moved. The move was done in two stages, from the airport site to the edge of Hanlan's Point where they spent the winter, then on to Sunfish Island, since renamed Algonquin Island, where they still stand. The bridge leading over the lagoon to Algonquin was rebuilt in 1998 in order that larger service vehicles, up to twenty-one tons (the old bridge was limited to just five ton vehicles) can access the Algonquin Island community.

  * The QUEEN CITY YACHT CLUB (QCYC) (180) is located at the extreme east end of Algonquin Island. This organization began in 1889 and first met in a small hut adjacent to the Queen's Wharf not far from the foot of Bathurst Street. It had several other mainland locations until the collapse of the York Street clubhouse into Toronto Bay on July 12, 1920, expedited the members' decision to move to Sunfish Island over on the Island. An interesting feature of the QCYC's Algonquin Island site is the use of the large iron hull of the former passenger steamer *Rapids Queen* as a breakwater. *Rapids Queen* was built in Chester, Pennsylvania in 1892 and launched on the Delaware River as the passenger steamer *Columbian*. In 1905, she was renamed *Brockville* and four years later, *Rapids Queen*. For the next three decades, she thrilled countless thousands of passengers as she "shot" the St. Lawrence River rapids between Prescott and Montreal. In 1939, *Rapids Queen* was sold, her superstructure removed, and she was converted into the utilitarian scow C.D. 110. The hull was purchased many years ago and towed to the present Algonquin Island site, where it has been positioned as a breakwater to protect the sandy QCYC beaches from erosion. Look, the ferry boat's just arriving at the dock. Time to return to the big city across the bay. Hope you've had fun!

## End of Walk Three

## Alphabetical Reference

Numbers indicate the location number for each site, as represented on the maps.